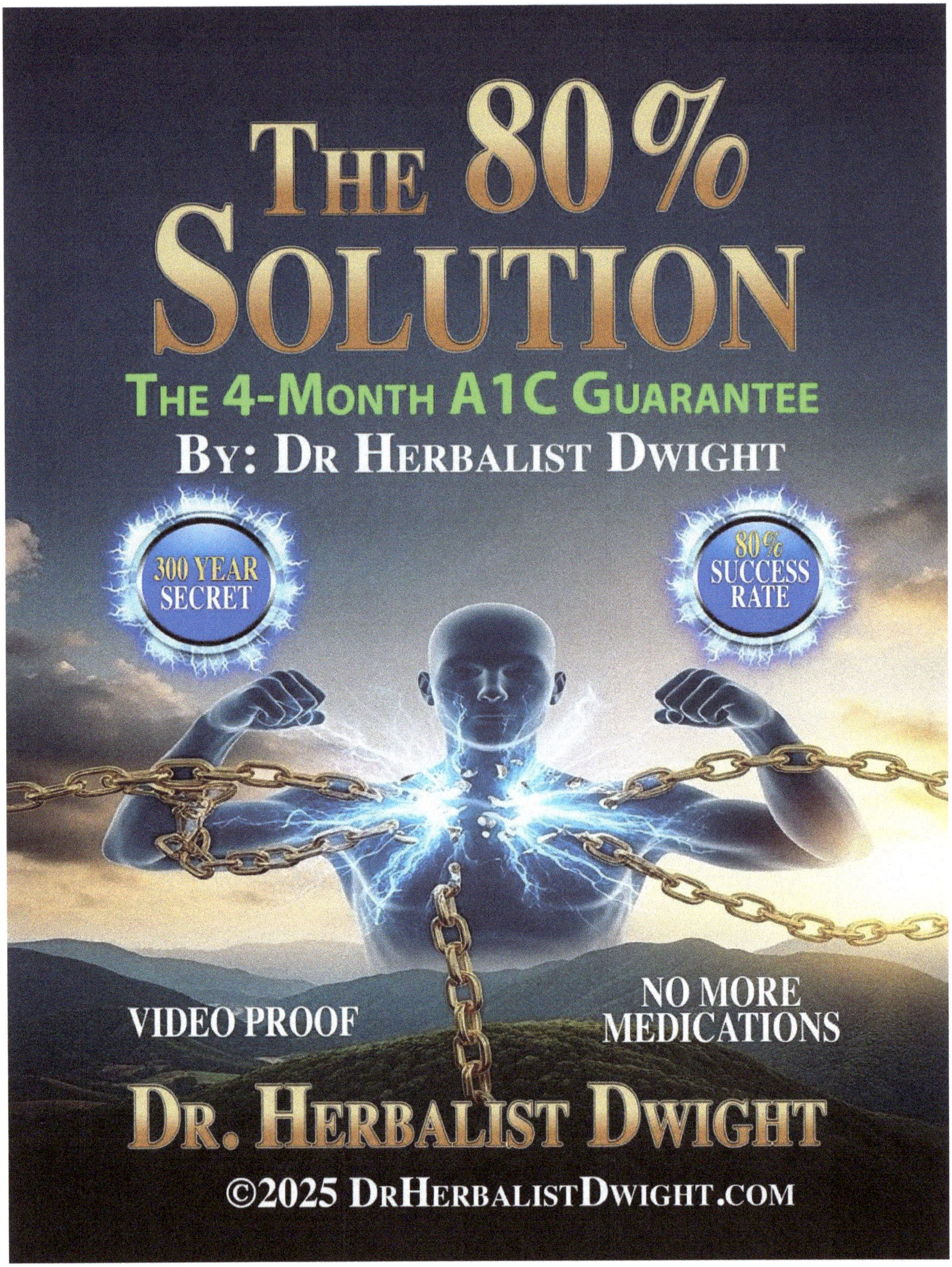

THE 80% SOLUTION
THE 4-MONTH A1C GUARANTEE
BY: DR HERBALIST DWIGHT
300 YEAR SECRET
80% SUCCESS RATE
VIDEO PROOF
NO MORE MEDICATIONS
DR. HERBALIST DWIGHT
©2025 DRHERBALISTDWIGHT.COM

THE 80% SOLUTION: THE 4-MONTH A1C GUARANTEE

Published by: Dr. Herbalist Dwight
Website: Drherbalistdwight.com
Email: info@drherbalistdwight.com
Phone: +1 307-922-8005

First Edition: 2025

ISBN: 979-8-9999920-0-0

IMPORTANT MEDICAL DISCLAIMER

This book is intended for educational and informational purposes only and should not be considered medical advice. The information contained herein is based on the author's personal experience, research, and traditional healing practices passed down through generations.

The statements in this book have not been evaluated by the Food and Drug Administration (FDA). The protocols, supplements, and dietary recommendations described in this book are not intended to diagnose, treat, cure, or prevent any disease.

Always consult with a qualified healthcare professional before making any changes to your diabetes medications, diet, or treatment plan. Never discontinue prescribed medications without proper medical supervision.

Individual results may vary. While the author reports an 80% success rate with the Sweet Blood Protocol, your individual results may differ based on various factors, including but not limited to: current health status, length of diabetes diagnosis, compliance with the protocol, other health conditions, medications, age, and lifestyle factors.

The author and publisher disclaim any liability for adverse effects arising from the use or application of the information contained in this book.

TRADITIONAL MEDICINE DISCLAIMER

The healing protocols described in this book are based on traditional Caribbean Maroon healing practices that have been passed down through over 300 years of ancestral knowledge. These traditional approaches have not been subjected to modern clinical trials as defined by conventional medical standards.

Traditional healing wisdom should complement, not replace, conventional medical care. Work with healthcare providers who are knowledgeable about both traditional and conventional approaches to diabetes management.

TESTIMONIAL DISCLAIMER

All client success stories and testimonials presented in this book represent real individuals who have used the Sweet Blood Protocol. However, these results are not typical and should not be expected by every reader.

Individual results will vary based on numerous factors. The testimonials are provided for educational purposes only and do not guarantee similar outcomes for other individuals.

The A1C results mentioned in testimonials were achieved under the supervision of healthcare providers and should not be attempted without proper medical oversight.

SUPPLEMENT AND HERBAL DISCLAIMER

The herbal supplements and natural remedies mentioned in this book are generally recognized as safe when used as directed. However:

- **Consult your healthcare provider** before starting any new supplement regimen
- **Inform your doctor** of all supplements you are taking
- **Be aware of potential interactions** with prescription medications
- **Discontinue use** if you experience any adverse reactions
- **Pregnant and nursing women** should consult healthcare providers before use

The author and publisher are not responsible for adverse reactions to supplements or herbs mentioned in this book.

DIETARY DISCLAIMER

The dietary recommendations in this book are based on traditional healing principles and the author's clinical experience. These recommendations:

- These are **general guidelines** and may not be suitable for everyone
- Should be **adapted to individual needs** and health conditions
- **May require modification** for people with food allergies or sensitivities
- Should be **discussed with healthcare providers,** especially for those with multiple health conditions

The author and publisher disclaim responsibility for any adverse effects resulting from dietary changes made based on this book.

CONSULTATION DISCLAIMER

The free 15-minute consultation offered in this book is for **educational purposes only** and does not constitute medical advice or create a doctor-patient relationship.

- Consultations are **informational discussions** about traditional healing approaches
- **Not a substitute for professional medical care**
- **Individual protocol recommendations** should be reviewed with your healthcare provider
- **No guarantee of results** from consultation recommendations

LIABILITY LIMITATION

To the fullest extent permitted by law, the author and publisher shall not be liable for any damages, including but not limited to direct, indirect, incidental, consequential, or punitive damages arising from the use of this book or the information contained herein.

By reading this book, you acknowledge that you understand these disclaimers and agree to use the information at your own risk.

CONTACT INFORMATION

For questions about this book or the Sweet Blood Protocol:

Dr. Herbalist Dwight LLC
Website: drherbalistdwight.com
Email: info@drherbalistdwight.com
Phone: +1 307-922-8005

Free 15-Minute Consultation: Dr Herbalist Dwight

ACKNOWLEDGMENTS

This book is dedicated to the ancestral wisdom of Queen Nanny and the Maroon healers of Jamaica's Blue Mountains, whose 300-year legacy of healing continues to transform lives today.

Special gratitude to the thousands of clients who have trusted this ancient wisdom and proven that diabetes reversal is possible through natural healing.

Printed in the United States of America

Contents

THE 80% SOLUTION: THE 4-MONTH A1C GUARANTEE

FOREWORD

"In the misty Blue Mountains of Jamaica, where my ancestors, the Maroons, fought for freedom, they also fought for something even more precious – the knowledge to heal. This book carries that 300-year legacy forward, offering you the same freedom from diabetes that has transformed thousands of lives."

Dr. Herbalist Dwight, Master Herbalist, Descendant of Queen Nanny's Maroon Lineage

INTRODUCTION:
THE CHOICE IS YOURS

Right now, as you read these words, you stand at a crossroads.

Down one path lies the conventional approach to diabetes – a lifetime of medications, blood sugar monitoring, dietary restrictions, and the constant fear of complications. It's the path of management, not healing. The path where diabetes "has no cure."

Down the other path lies something your doctor has never told you about – a 300-year-old Caribbean healing protocol that has helped over 80% of people completely reverse their diabetes in just 4 months.

I am Dr. Herbalist Dwight, and I've spent over 65 years mastering the ancient healing arts passed down through Queen Nanny's legendary Maroon lineage in Jamaica's Blue Mountains. What I'm about to share with you isn't theory – it's proven results from real people whose lives have been transformed.

The 80% Solution isn't just a catchy title; it's a practical approach to achieving success. It's a guarantee.

In the next 4 months, following the Sweet Blood Protocol detailed in this book, you have an 80% chance of:

- Reducing your A1C to normal levels (below 5.7)
- Eliminating or dramatically reducing diabetes medications
- Experiencing stable blood sugar throughout the day
- Regaining energy, vitality, and confidence in your health

But here's what makes this different from every other diabetes book you've read: **Every success story in this book is video-verified.** These aren't anonymous testimonials or cherry-picked results. These are real people with real names, real faces, and real medical documentation of their transformation.

Meet just a few of them:

- **Rufus**: A1C dropped from 10.6 to 4.8, insulin-free for 3 years
- **Kim**: A1C fell from 10.4 to 5.7, off metformin for 3 years
- **Angela**: A1C reduced from 9.8 to 5.6, completely drug-free
- **Doretha**: A1C dropped from 10.2 to 6.0 in just 3 weeks

Their stories, along with those of dozens of others, are documented throughout this book, accompanied by links to their video testimonials.

Why This Protocol Works When Others Fail

The Sweet Blood Protocol addresses what conventional medicine ignores – the root cause of diabetes. While pharmaceutical approaches focus on managing symptoms, this 300-year-old wisdom targets the underlying metabolic dysfunction that creates diabetes in the first place.

This isn't about restricting your life. It's about restoring your body's natural ability to regulate blood sugar, just as it was designed to do.

Your 4-Month Journey Starts Here.

This book is your comprehensive guide to achieving diabetes freedom. You'll discover:

- The exact herbal formulations used by Caribbean healers for centuries
- The Four Pillars that form the foundation of metabolic healing
- Daily protocols for morning, midday, evening, and sleep optimization
- The specific foods that heal versus those that harm
- A week-by-week transformation timeline
- How to maintain your results for life

A Personal Invitation

Before we begin this journey together, I want to offer you something that no other diabetes book can – a personal consultation with me.

Schedule Your FREE 15-Minute Consultation.

During this call, we'll discuss your specific situation and how the Sweet Blood Protocol can be customized for your unique needs.

The Choice Is Still Yours

You can close this book right now and continue down the path of diabetes management – the injections, the medications, the complications, the fear.

Or you can turn the page and discover what thousands of people already know: diabetes is not a life sentence. It's a condition that can be reversed when you address the root cause with the proper knowledge and understanding.

The 300-year-old wisdom of my ancestors awaits you.

The choice is yours.

Dr. Herbalist Dwight Master Herbalist,

Chapter 1
"THE MIRACLE THAT CHANGED EVERYTHING "
(Zack's 7-day story)

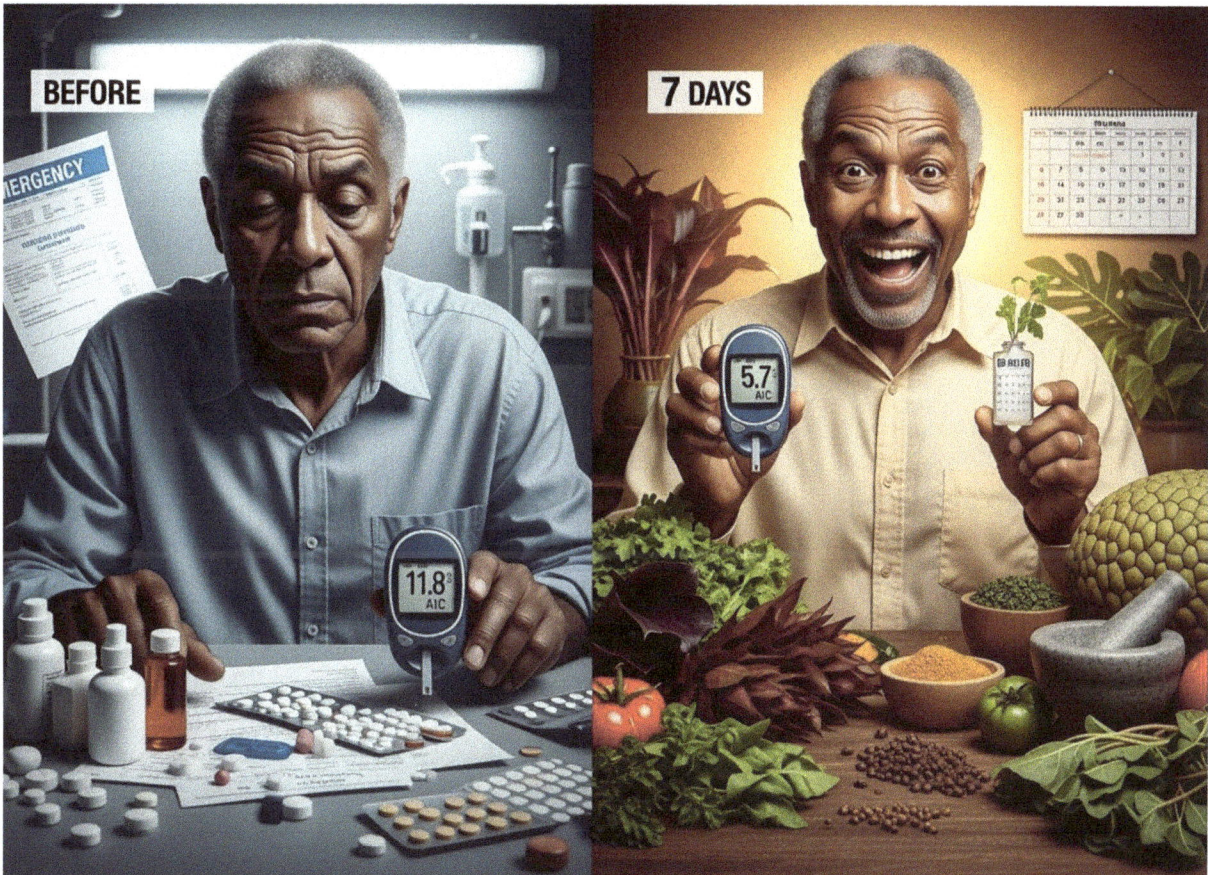

The Day Everything Changed: Zack's 7-Day Miracle

The phone rang at 3:47 AM. After 65 years of healing people, I've learned that desperate calls come at desperate hours.

"Dr. Dwight?" The voice was shaking. "My name is Zack. I'm... I'm dying. My A1C is 11.8. The doctors say I have maybe weeks before my organs start shutting down. They want to put me on insulin immediately, but I heard about you from my neighbor. She said, "You do miracles.""

I sat up in bed, fully awake. A1C of 11.8 - that's not just diabetes, that's a medical emergency. Most herbalists would advise him to go straight to the hospital. But I've seen this before, in the mountains of Jamaica, in the villages of Africa, in the healing centers of Asia. When death knocks, sometimes ancient wisdom answers.

"Zack," I said quietly, "what if I told you you could be completely free from diabetes? Would you trust me?"

Silence. Then a broken whisper: "I'll try anything."

Day 1: The Foundation Zack arrived at my clinic looking like death itself - gray skin, sunken eyes, hands shaking from blood sugar chaos. I began with the first pillar of the Sweet Blood Protocol: blood purification using herbs my mother taught me in Queen Nanny's mountains.

"This tastes terrible," he grimaced, drinking the bitter tea.

"Terrible taste, miraculous results," I smiled. "Your ancestors knew this. Your body remembers."

Day 3: The Turning Point Zack called me, voice different. "Dr. Dwight, something's happening. I woke up without that fog in my head. My hands aren't shaking."

I checked his glucose: 180 mg/dL. Still high, but dropping fast. The 300-year protocol was working.

Day 5: The Acceleration "I can't believe this," Zack whispered, staring at his glucose meter. "142. I haven't seen numbers this low in years."

The four pillars were working in perfect harmony - blood purification, pancreatic restoration, insulin sensitivity reset, and metabolic rebalancing. Just as they had for three centuries in my family line.

Day 7: The Miracle Zack walked into my office a different man. Bright eyes, steady hands, glowing skin. He held up his A1C test results with tears streaming down his face.

"5.7," he whispered. "From 11.8 to 5.7 in seven days. The doctors are calling it impossible. They're demanding to know what I did."

I smiled, thinking of my great-grandmother's words: "When the body remembers its original design, healing happens faster than the mind can believe."

The Ripple Effect. That was three years ago. Zack is still diabetes-free, still medication-free, still sharing his story with anyone who'll listen. His "impossible" 7-day transformation became the foundation for helping thousands more discover that diabetes isn't a life sentence - it's a wake-up call.

The Sweet Blood Protocol that saved Zack's life in 7 days typically takes 4 months for most people. But Zack's story proves that when ancient wisdom meets desperate faith, miracles still happen.

Some people need 4 months. Some need 7 days. Everyone deserves freedom.

That's the power of 300-year-old healing wisdom - it doesn't just manage diabetes, it eliminates it entirely.

Ready to write your own miracle story?

CHAPTER 2
THE FAILURE OF CONVENTIONAL DIABETES CARE

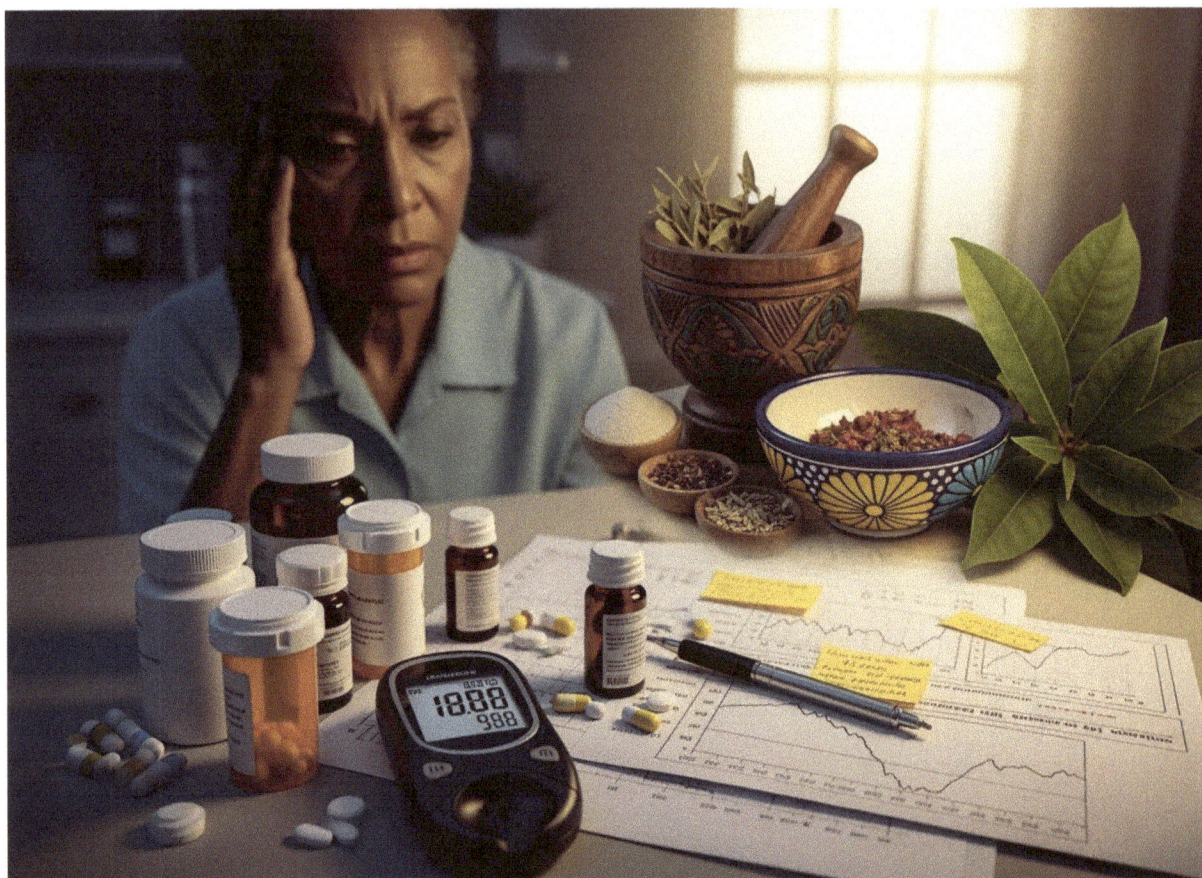

"The definition of insanity is doing the same thing over and over again and expecting different results. Yet this is exactly what conventional diabetes care asks you to do."

Michele sat in her endocrinologist's office, tears streaming down her face. After 15 years of "managing" her Type 2 diabetes, her A1C had climbed to 9.8. Her doctor was recommending insulin – the final step in what felt like a slow march toward inevitable complications.

"But I've done everything you told me," Michele pleaded. "I take my metformin religiously. I check my blood sugar multiple times a day. I follow the diabetic diet. Why is it getting worse?"

Her doctor's response was the same script millions of people with diabetes hear: "Diabetes is a progressive disease. We need to add more medication."

Three months later, Michele found my protocol. Today, her A1C is 5.4, and she's completely medication-free.

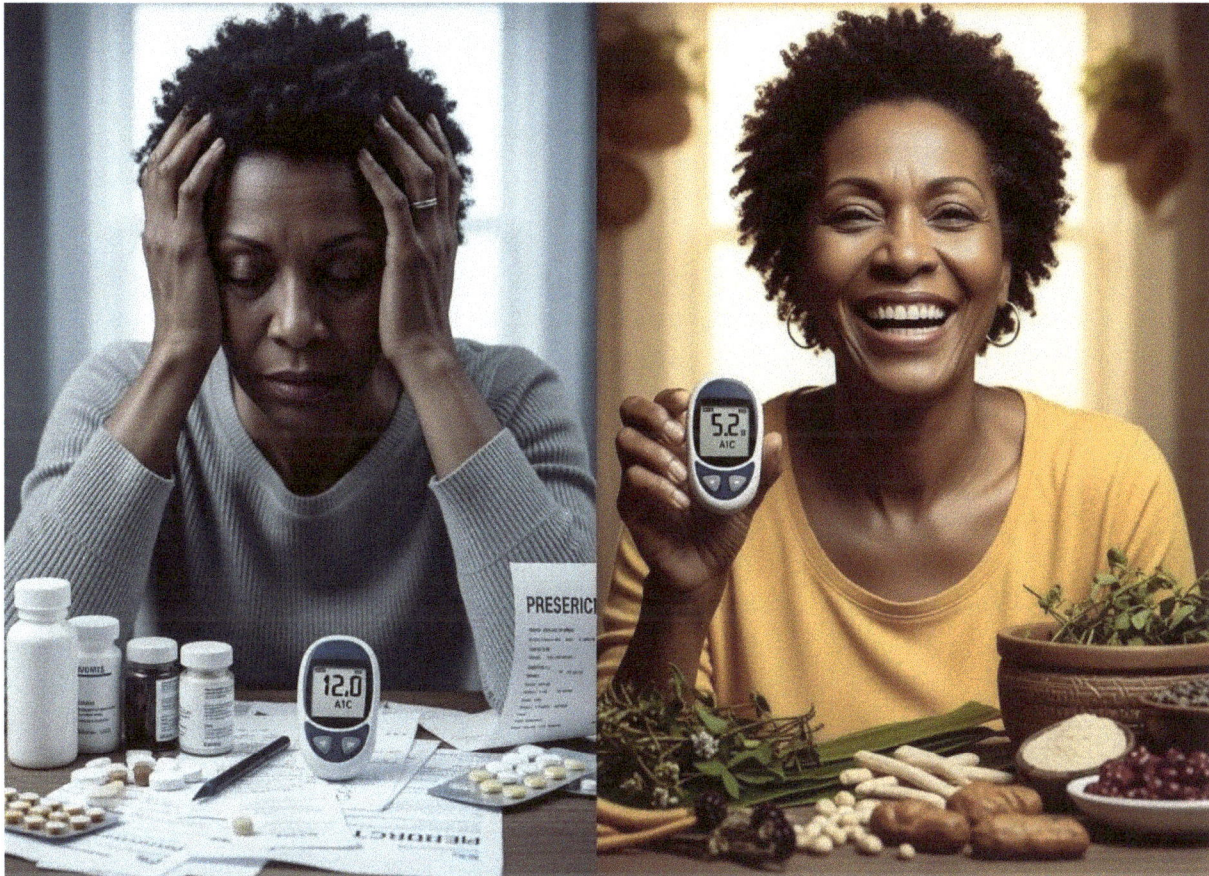

Her transformation is documented in [the video testimonial, "Michele's Story."](#)

The Trillion-Dollar Failure

The statistics are staggering and shameful:

- **37.3 million Americans** have diabetes
- **96 million Americans** have prediabetes
- **$327 billion** is spent annually on diabetes care
- **Diabetes cases have TRIPLED** in the past 30 years

Despite spending more money than ever before, diabetes rates continue to skyrocket. Why?

Because conventional medicine treats diabetes backwards.

The Symptom Management Trap

Modern diabetes care operates on a fundamentally flawed premise: that diabetes is an incurable, progressive disease that can only be "managed." This approach focuses entirely on controlling blood sugar levels through external means – medications, insulin, and dietary restrictions – while completely ignoring the underlying metabolic dysfunction.

It's like trying to fix a leaky roof by placing buckets on the floor. You might catch the water, but you're not fixing the hole.

Here's what conventional diabetes care actually does:

1. **Masks the problem** with medications instead of addressing root causes
2. **Creates medication dependence** that often worsens over time
3. **Ignores metabolic healing** in favor of symptom suppression
4. **Focuses on numbers** rather than overall health restoration
5. **Accepts complications** as inevitable rather than preventable

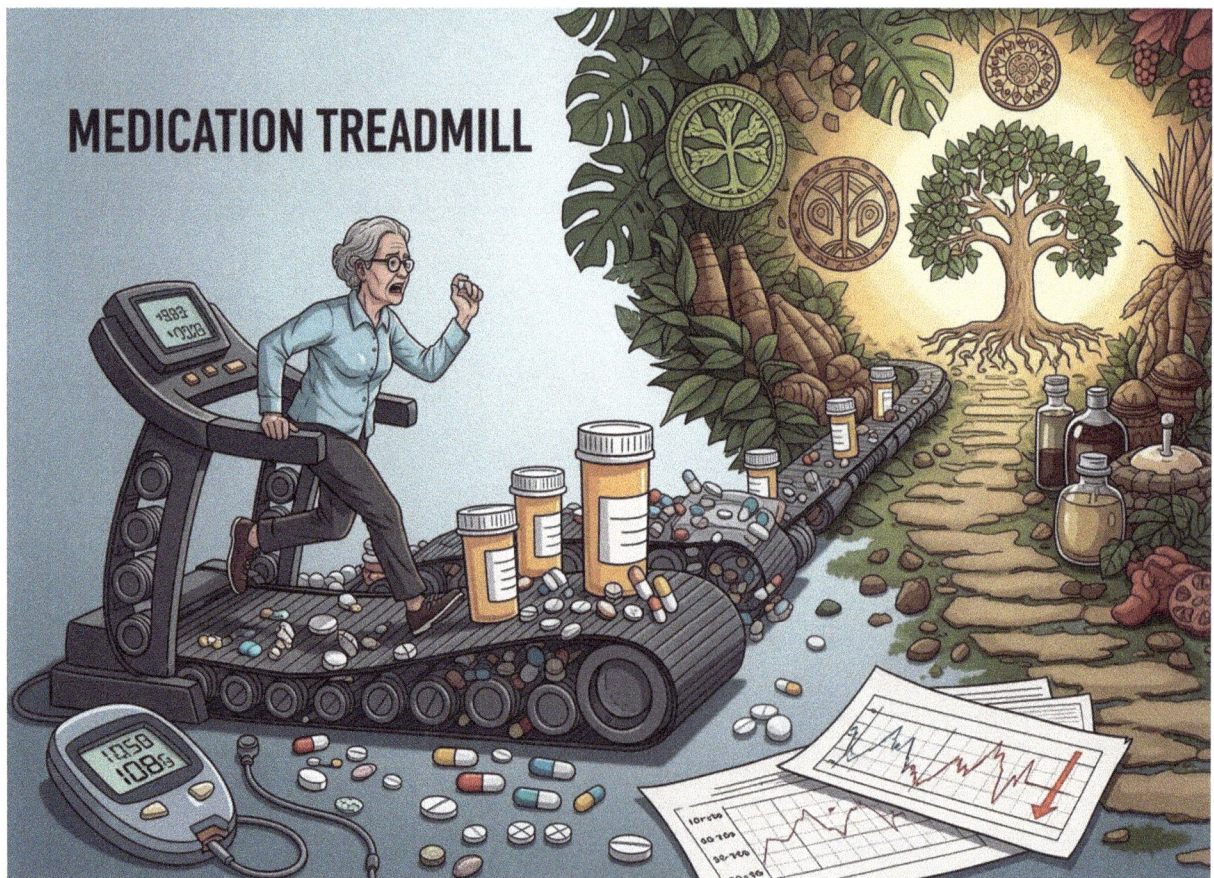

The standard diabetes treatment protocol follows a predictable, devastating pattern:

Stage 1: Diagnosis

- Metformin prescribed
- "Lifestyle changes" recommended (usually ineffective generic advice)
- Patient told diabetes is "manageable but not curable"

Stage 2: Progression

- Blood sugar control worsens despite medication

- Additional drugs added (sulfonylureas, SGLT2 inhibitors, etc.)
- Side effects begin to compound

Stage 3: Intensification

- Multiple medications required
- Insulin introduced
- Patient accepts "progressive disease" narrative

Stage 4: Complications

- Neuropathy, retinopathy, and nephropathy develop
- More specialists added to the care team
- Quality of life significantly diminished

The Hidden Truth About Diabetes Medications

What your doctor doesn't tell you about diabetes medications:

Metformin:

- Depletes Vitamin B12, leading to neuropathy
- Causes digestive issues in up to 25% of users
- May actually worsen insulin resistance over time

Sulfonylureas:

- Force exhausted pancreatic cells to work harder
- Increase risk of hypoglycemia and weight gain
- May accelerate pancreatic beta cell death

Insulin:

- Promotes fat storage and weight gain
- Creates a cycle of increasing insulin resistance
- Requires constant dose adjustments

SGLT2 Inhibitors:

- Risk of diabetic ketoacidosis
- Increased infections and amputations
- Kidney and cardiovascular concerns

Why the "Diabetic Diet" Fails

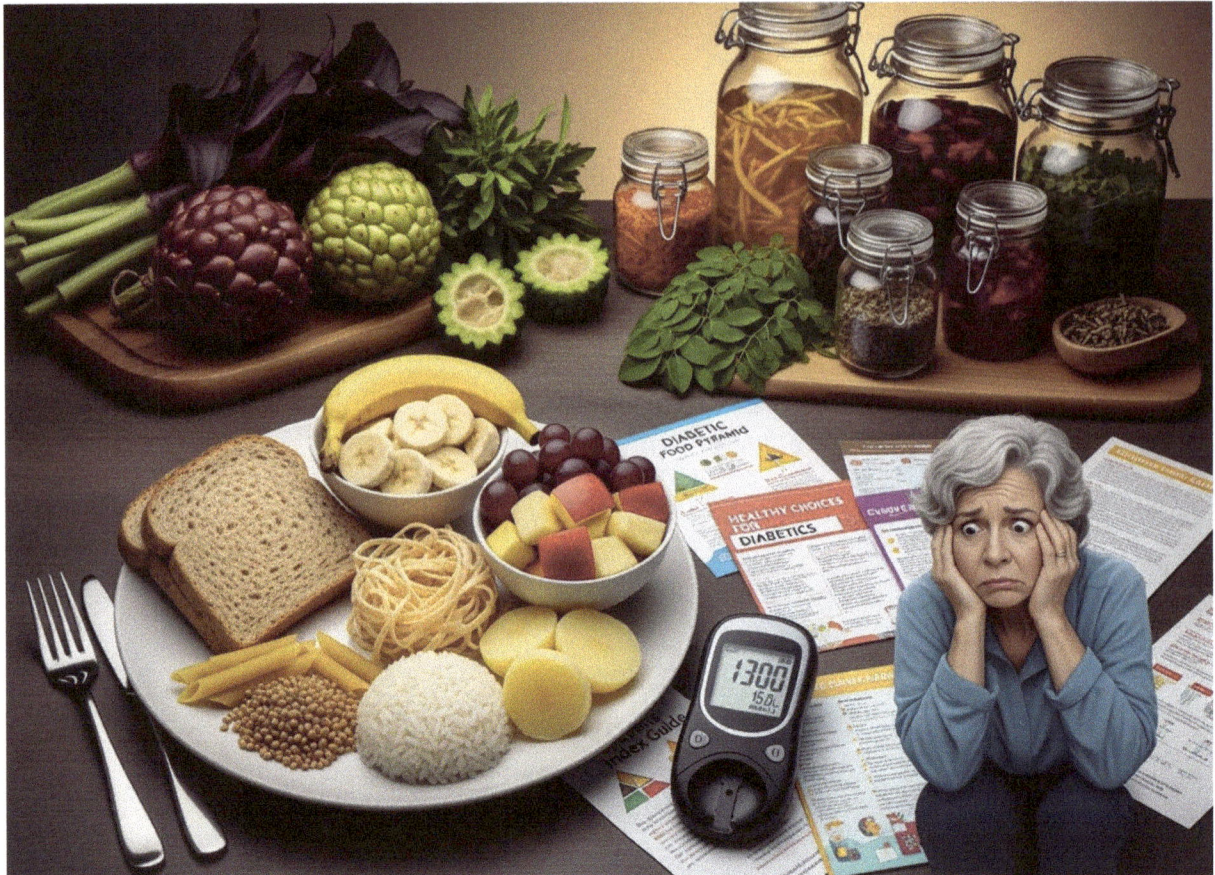

The standard diabetic diet recommended by most healthcare providers is nutritionally bankrupt and metabolically harmful. Based on the outdated food pyramid, it typically recommends:

- **60% carbohydrates** (the very macronutrient that raises blood sugar)
- **Processed "diabetic" foods** loaded with artificial sweeteners
- **Low-fat recommendations** that increase sugar cravings
- **Frequent small meals** that keep insulin constantly elevated

Is it any wonder that following this advice leads to worsening diabetes?

The Real Success Stories They Don't Want You to See

While conventional medicine claims that diabetes reversal is impossible, thousands of people are proving them wrong by using natural protocols, like the one detailed in this book.

Rufus's Story: When Rufus came to me, his A1C was 10.6 and climbing despite maximum doses of metformin and insulin. His doctors wanted to add yet another medication. Instead, Rufus chose the Sweet Blood Protocol.

Within 4 months:

- A1C dropped to 5.8
- Completely off all diabetes medications
- Lost 33 pounds naturally
- Energy levels restored

Three years later, Rufus remains diabetes-free. And A1C is 4.8. **Watch Rufus's Complete Transformation Video**

Kim's Breakthrough: Kim's A1C of 10.4 prompted her doctors to prepare for insulin therapy. She was told her pancreas was "burned out" and that medication would be lifelong.

The Sweet Blood Protocol proved them wrong:

- A1C normalized to 6.1 in 4 months
- Off metformin for over 3 years
- No longer considers herself diabetic
- Helps others find the same freedom

See Kim's Medical Records and Testimonial

The Paradigm Shift

The difference between conventional diabetes care and the Sweet Blood Protocol is the difference between:

Conventional Approach:

- Manages symptoms
- Accepts progression
- Creates dependence
- Focuses on blood sugar numbers
- Ignores root causes

Sweet Blood Protocol:

- Heals metabolically
- Reverses progression
- Restores independence
- Focuses on overall health
- Addresses root causes

The Economic Incentive Problem

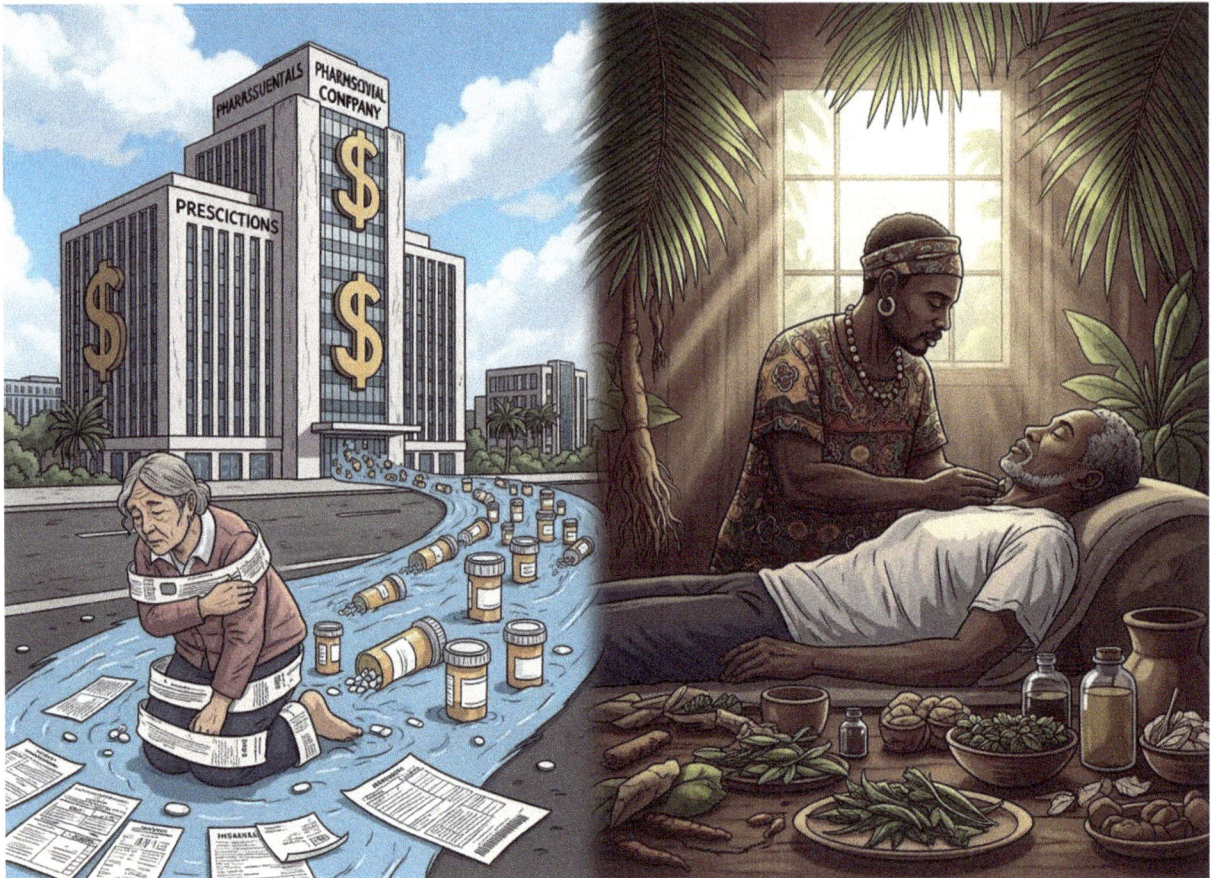

Here's an uncomfortable truth: there's no financial incentive for the medical establishment to cure diabetes. A cured diabetic is a lost customer.

Consider the lifetime value of a diabetic patient:

- **Average annual cost:** $16,752
- **Average lifespan with diabetes:** 20-30 years
- **Lifetime value:** $335,000-$500,000 per patient

The diabetes industry generates over $327 billion in annual revenue. Curing diabetes would eliminate this revenue stream overnight.

This isn't a conspiracy – it's simple economics. The system is designed to manage disease, not cure it.

Your Doctor's Limitations

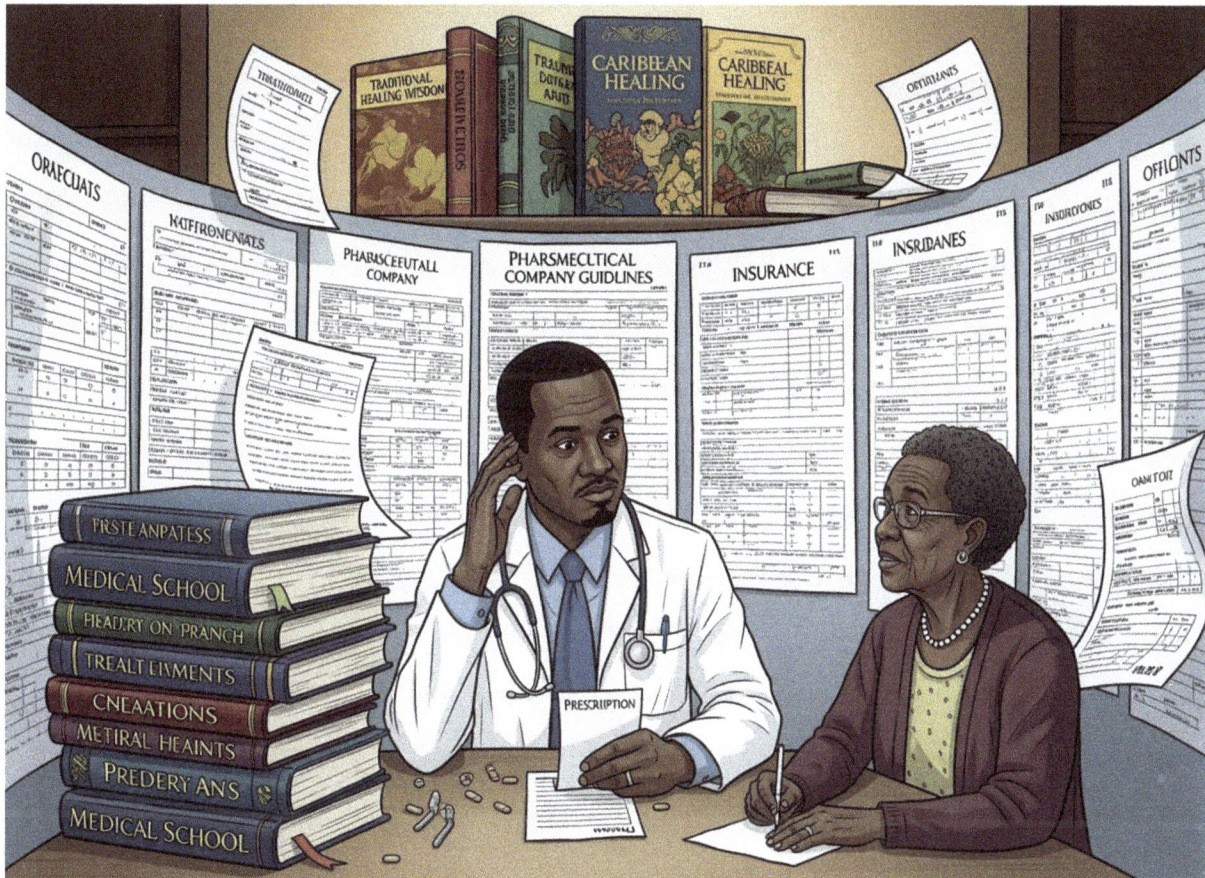

Most physicians are genuinely caring people who want to help their patients. However, they're trapped within a system that:

- Provides only 4-6 hours of nutrition education in medical school
- Focuses on pharmaceutical interventions
- Penalizes "alternative" approaches
- Operates on 15-minute appointment schedules
- Lacks training in metabolic healing

Your doctor isn't withholding a cure – they simply don't know about it.

The 300-Year Alternative

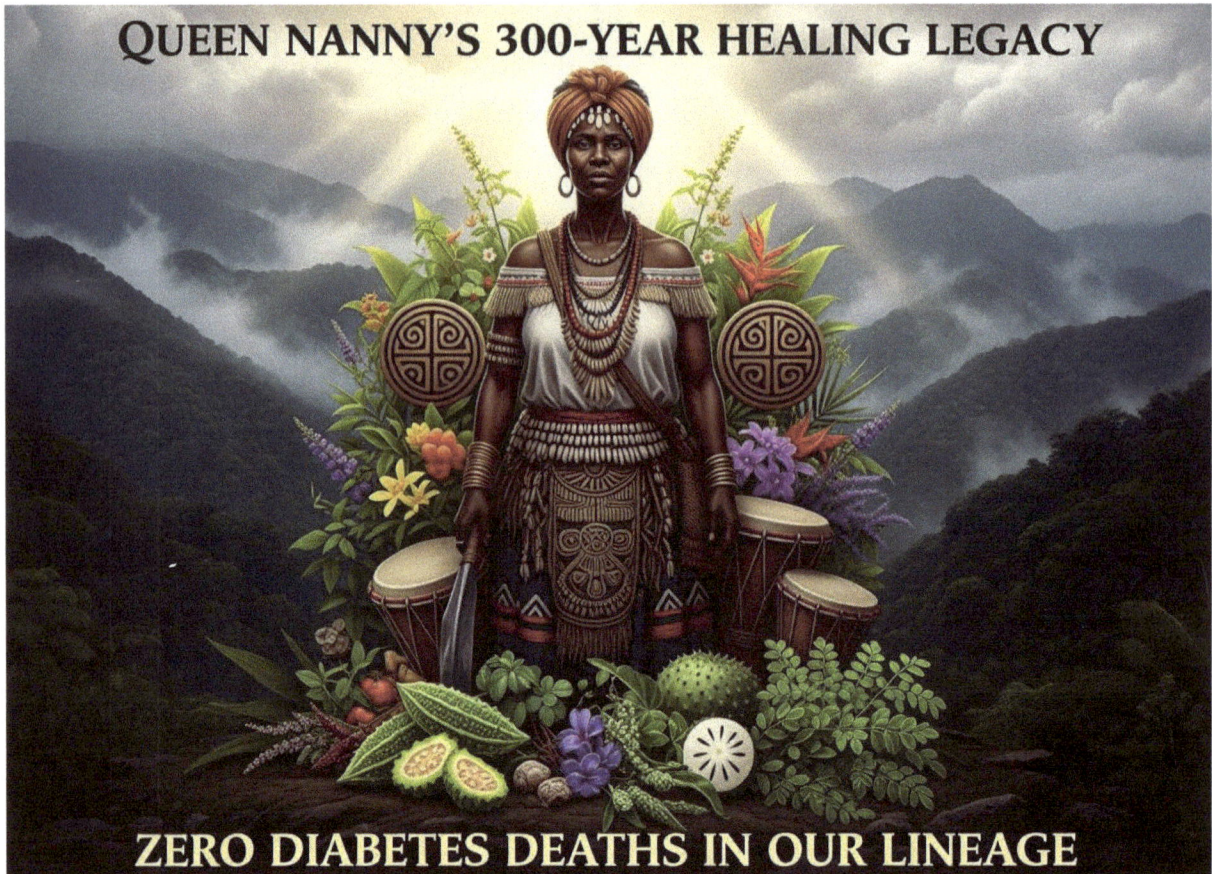

QUEEN NANNY'S 300-YEAR HEALING LEGACY

ZERO DIABETES DEATHS IN OUR LINEAGE

While modern medicine has failed diabetics for decades, Caribbean healers have been successfully reversing diabetes for centuries using the Sweet Blood Protocol.

This isn't folk medicine or wishful thinking. It's a systematic approach to metabolic healing that addresses diabetes at its source – insulin resistance and pancreatic dysfunction.

The protocol you'll learn in this book has:

- **300 years of traditional use**
- **80% success rate in clinical application**
- **Thousands of documented reversals**
- **Video-verified testimonials**
- **No harmful side effects**

Breaking Free from the System

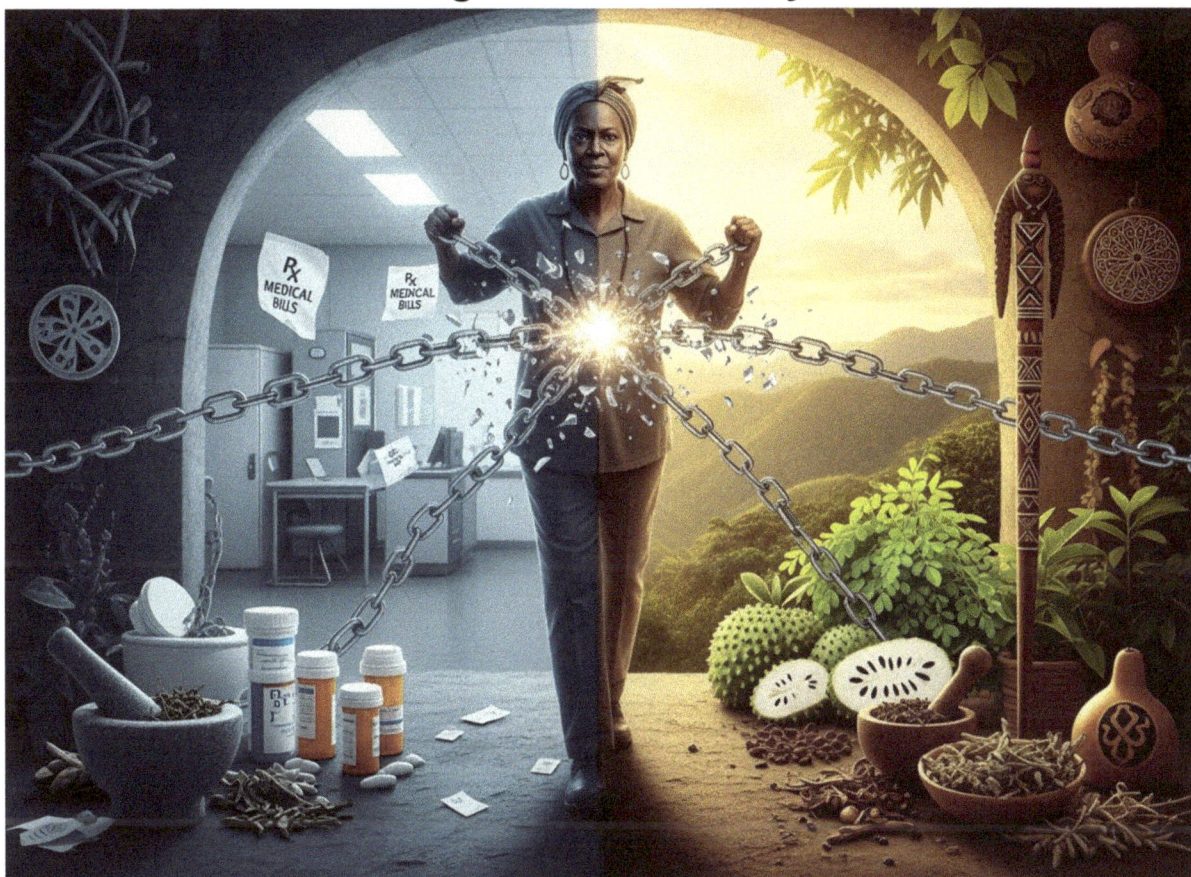

The first step in reversing your diabetes is recognizing that the conventional approach has not worked for you. It's not your fault that medications haven't worked. It's not your fault that your diabetes has progressed despite following medical advice.

The system is broken, but you don't have to remain broken with it.

What's Coming Next

In the following chapters, you'll discover:

- The fascinating history of the Sweet Blood Protocol (Chapter 2)
- Real success stories with video documentation (Chapter 3)
- The exact protocol that reverses diabetes (Chapter 4)
- Your daily implementation guide (Chapters 5-8)
- The foods that heal vs. harm (Chapters 9-10)
- Your 4-month transformation timeline (Chapter 11)
- How to maintain your results for life (Chapter 12)

Your Free Consultation Awaits

Before we delve deeper into the protocol, I would like to personally invite you to experience what personalized diabetes reversal guidance is like.

[Schedule Your FREE 15-Minute Consultation.](#)

During this call, we'll discuss:

- Your current diabetes situation
- Which aspects of the Sweet Blood Protocol are most relevant for you
- How to customize the approach for your specific needs
- Any questions you have about natural diabetes reversal

The Choice Remains Yours

You now understand why conventional diabetes care has not been effective for you. The question is: what will you do with this knowledge?

You can return to the medication treadmill, accepting "management" as your fate.

Or you can turn the page and discover the 300-year-old wisdom that has freed thousands from diabetes forever.

The choice is yours.

In the next chapter, we'll journey back to the misty Blue Mountains of Jamaica, where Queen Nanny's Maroons developed the healing protocols that would change everything...

CHAPTER 3
THE 300-YEAR HERITAGE OF HEALING

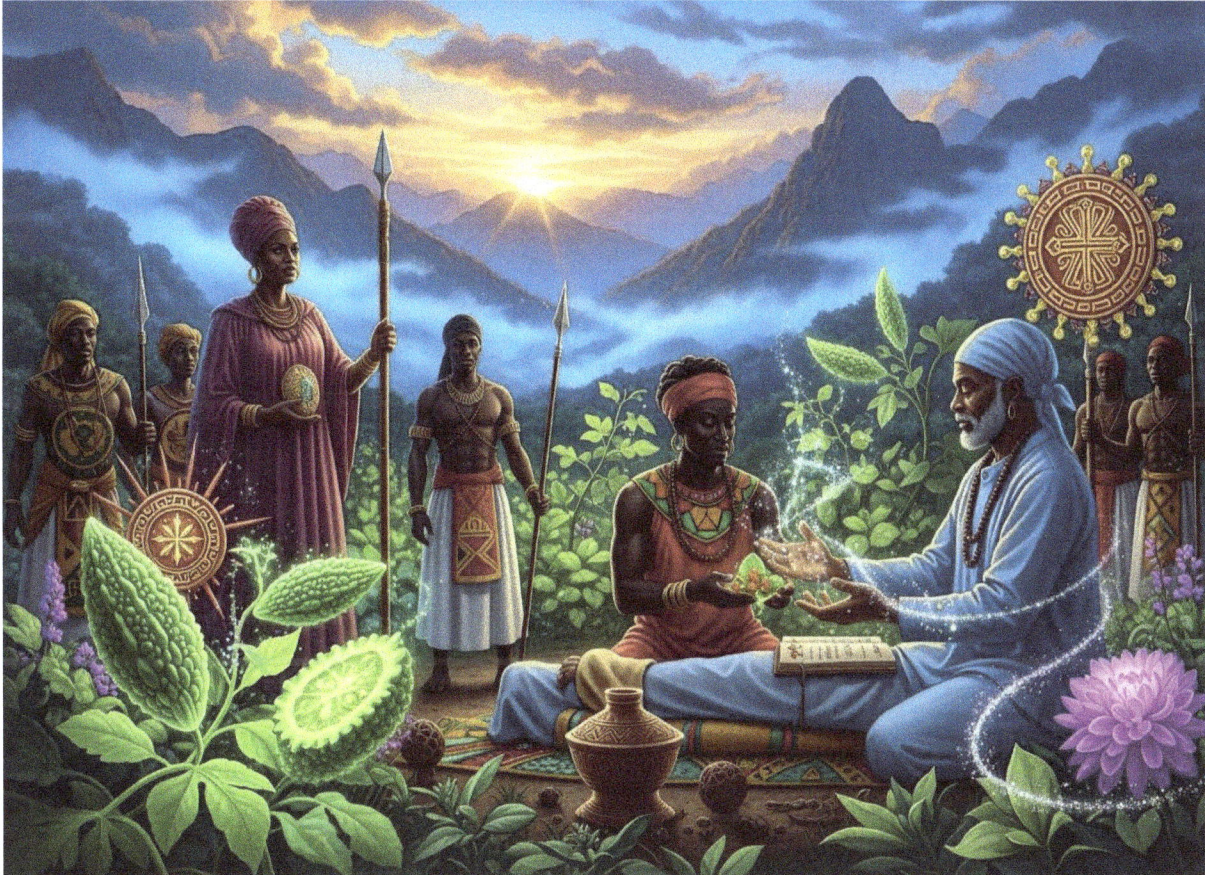

"In the mist-covered peaks of Jamaica's Blue Mountains, where my ancestors fought for freedom, they discovered something more valuable than gold – the knowledge to heal the body's deepest ailments."

The year was 1720. Queen Nanny, the legendary Maroon leader, stood in her mountain stronghold watching British soldiers retreat once again from her impenetrable fortress. But this victory wasn't won with muskets or machetes – it was won with knowledge.

The same healing wisdom that kept her warriors strong and healthy in the harsh mountain terrain would eventually become the Sweet Blood Protocol that has reversed diabetes in over 80% of the people who've used it.

I am the living bridge between that ancient wisdom and your modern healing.

The Maroon Legacy

Most people are familiar with the Maroons as fierce warriors who successfully resisted British colonization for over 80 years. What they don't know is that the Maroons were also master healers, carrying forward a sophisticated understanding of plant medicine that had been passed down through generations.

My lineage traces directly back to Queen Nanny herself. For 300 years, this healing knowledge has been carefully preserved and passed from grandmother to granddaughter, from master herbalist to apprentice, through an unbroken chain of wisdom that now reaches you through this book.

The Original Diabetes Epidemic

Even in the 1700s, the Maroons experienced what is now known as Type 2 diabetes. They called it "sweet blood sickness" – a condition where the body's natural ability to process sugar became disrupted, leading to weakness, excessive thirst, and slow-healing wounds.

But unlike modern medicine, which treats diabetes as incurable, the Maroons understood it as a metabolic imbalance that could be corrected through specific plant medicines and lifestyle practices.

The protocol they developed wasn't just effective – it was transformative. Those who followed it didn't just manage their sweet blood sickness; they eliminated it entirely.

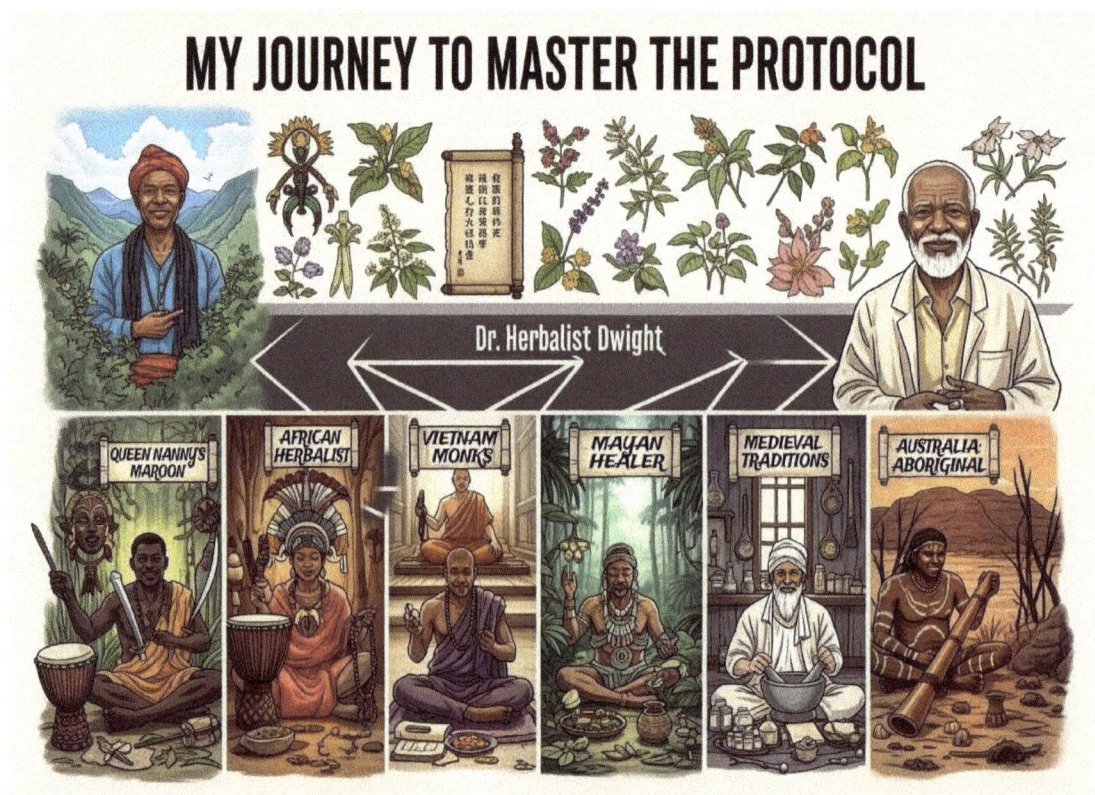

MY JOURNEY TO MASTER THE PROTOCOL

Dr. Herbalist Dwight

QUEEN NANNY'S MAROON · AFRICAN HERBALIST · VIETNAM MONKS · MAYAN HEALER · MEDIEVAL TRADITIONS · AUSTRALIA ABORIGINAL

My Journey to Master the Protocol

My education in this ancient art began before I could walk. In the Blue Mountains of Jamaica, surrounded by the same medicinal plants my ancestors used, I learned from my mother, now 102 years old and still a practicing master herbalist.

The Early Years (Ages 0-11): Every morning began with plant identification walks through the mountain forests. I learned to recognize healing herbs not just by sight, but by smell, texture, and even the sound they made in the wind. My mother would quiz me constantly:

"What plant stops the sugar sickness?" "Which combination heals the blood?" "How do you prepare the morning medicine?"

By age 8, I could identify over 200 medicinal plants and prepare basic healing formulations. By 11, I was already helping treat neighbors with various ailments, including several cases of sweet blood sickness.

The Global Education (Ages 12-65): When my family moved to New York, I thought my higher education was over. I was wrong – it was just beginning on a global scale.

Over the next 50+ years, I would travel to six continents, studying with traditional healers in:

- **Africa:** Learning from Sangomas and traditional doctors about blood purification
- **Asia:** Studying with Ayurvedic masters and Traditional Chinese Medicine practitioners
- **Europe:** Discovering medieval herbal traditions and modern phytotherapy
- **Australia:** Learning from Aboriginal healers about desert plant medicines
- **Central America:** Mastering Mayan healing traditions in Belize
- **South America:** Studying with shamans and curanderos

Each tradition added layers of understanding to the original Maroon protocol, but the core remained unchanged – diabetes is a metabolic imbalance that can be healed through specific plant medicines and lifestyle practices.

The Sweet Blood Protocol Revealed

The protocol that has transformed thousands of lives is built on four fundamental principles discovered by my Maroon ancestors:

1. Blood Purification. Sweet blood sickness begins with toxic blood. The first step is always deep blood cleansing using specific Caribbean herbs that pull toxins from the bloodstream and restore proper circulation.

2. Pancreatic Restoration The pancreas isn't "burned out" as conventional medicine claims – it's overwhelmed and inflamed. Specific plants can help reduce inflammation and support the restoration of natural insulin production.

3. Insulin Sensitivity Reset. Insulin resistance is reversible when you know which plants restore cellular sensitivity to insulin. The Maroons identified several key herbs that act as natural metformin, but without the side effects.

4. Metabolic Rebalancing True healing requires rebalancing the entire metabolic system – liver function, adrenal health, thyroid optimization, and digestive restoration. The protocol addresses all of these simultaneously.

The Modern Validation

What my ancestors knew intuitively, modern science is now proving:

Recent Research Confirms:

- Bitter melon contains compounds that mimic insulin
- Cinnamon bark improves insulin sensitivity by up to 40%
- Gymnema sylvestre can regenerate pancreatic beta cells
- Chromium supplementation reduces A1C levels significantly
- Alpha-lipoic acid reverses diabetic neuropathy

But here's what science can't replicate – the synergistic combinations and specific preparations that make these plants maximally effective. That knowledge lives only in the traditional protocols passed down through my family.

Real Results from Real People

The Sweet Blood Protocol isn't theoretical. It's been tested and proven in thousands of real-world cases. Let me share just a few of the documented transformations:

Kim's Transformation: When Kim first contacted me, her A1C level was 10.4 and rising, despite taking the maximum dose of metformin. Her doctor was preparing to add insulin to her regimen.

"I was desperate," Kim recalls in her video testimonial. "I'd tried every diet, every medication adjustment. Nothing worked. I was resigned to a lifetime of increasing medications and decreasing health."

Within the first month on the Sweet Blood Protocol:

- Her morning blood sugars dropped from 280 to 140
- Energy levels began returning
- Sugar cravings disappeared
- Sleep quality improved dramatically

By month 4:

- A1C had normalized to 6.1
- Completely off metformin
- Lost 50 pounds naturally
- Felt better than she had in years

Three years later, Kim remains completely diabetes-free. Watch Kim's Complete Transformation Video

Rufus's Miracle: Rufus came to me with an A1C of 10.6, taking both metformin and insulin. His doctors had told him his pancreas was "burned out" and that he'd need increasing amounts of insulin for life.

The Sweet Blood Protocol proved them wrong:

Week 1: Blood sugar levels began to stabilize. Week 4: Insulin doses reduced by 50% Week 8: Completely off insulin. Week 16: A1C tested at 5.8 – completely normal

Three years later, Rufus has maintained his diabetes-free status with no medications. See Rufus's Video Story

The Preparation Process

The Sweet Blood Protocol isn't just about taking herbs – it's about preparing them correctly. This knowledge has been refined over the past 300 years to maximize bioavailability and therapeutic efficacy.

Traditional Preparation Methods:

Morning Decoction: Specific roots and barks are slow-simmered for exactly 45 minutes to extract water-soluble compounds while preserving heat-sensitive nutrients.

Midday Tincture: Alcohol-based extractions of leaves and flowers, prepared during specific lunar phases for maximum potency.

Evening Powder: Dried and ground herbs combined in precise ratios, taken with specific carrier foods to enhance absorption.

Monthly Cleanse: A 3-day intensive protocol using rare Caribbean herbs to reset the entire metabolic system.

Each preparation method serves a specific purpose in the overall healing process. This isn't random folk medicine – it's a sophisticated system of metabolic restoration.

Why This Protocol Succeeds Where Others Fail

The Sweet Blood Protocol succeeds because it addresses diabetes holistically:

Conventional Approach:

- Focuses only on blood sugar numbers
- Ignores underlying metabolic dysfunction
- Creates medication dependence
- Accepts disease progression as inevitable

Sweet Blood Protocol:

- Addresses root metabolic causes
- Restores natural body function
- Creates lasting independence from medications
- Reverses disease progression

The Living Tradition

This isn't ancient history – it's a living, breathing tradition that continues to evolve. My 102-year-old mother still practices in Jamaica, treating diabetes patients with the same protocols I use today.

When I established Mayan Botanicals in Belize, I continued this tradition, working with local Mayan healers who had their own versions of diabetes-healing protocols. The synergy between Caribbean Maroon wisdom and Mayan plant medicine has made the Sweet Blood Protocol even more effective.

Your Connection to This Heritage

When you begin the Sweet Blood Protocol, you're not just taking herbs – you're connecting with 300 years of healing wisdom. You're joining a lineage of people who refused to accept diabetes as a life sentence.

Every person who has reversed their diabetes using this protocol becomes part of this living tradition. They carry forward the knowledge that healing is possible, that the body can restore itself when given the right tools.

The Responsibility of Knowledge

With this knowledge comes responsibility. The Sweet Blood Protocol represents centuries of accumulated wisdom on naturally healing diabetes. It's not just information – it's a sacred trust passed down through generations of healers.

This is why every person who successfully uses the protocol has a responsibility to share their story, helping others understand that diabetes reversal is possible.

Your Personal Consultation

Before we delve deeper into the specific protocols, I would like to offer you the same personalized guidance that has helped thousands of people successfully manage their diabetes.

Schedule Your FREE 15-Minute Consultation

During this call, we'll discuss:

- Your specific diabetes situation and health history
- Which aspects of the Sweet Blood Protocol are most relevant for you
- How to customize the approach based on your current medications
- Any concerns or questions you have about natural diabetes reversal

The Bridge Between Worlds

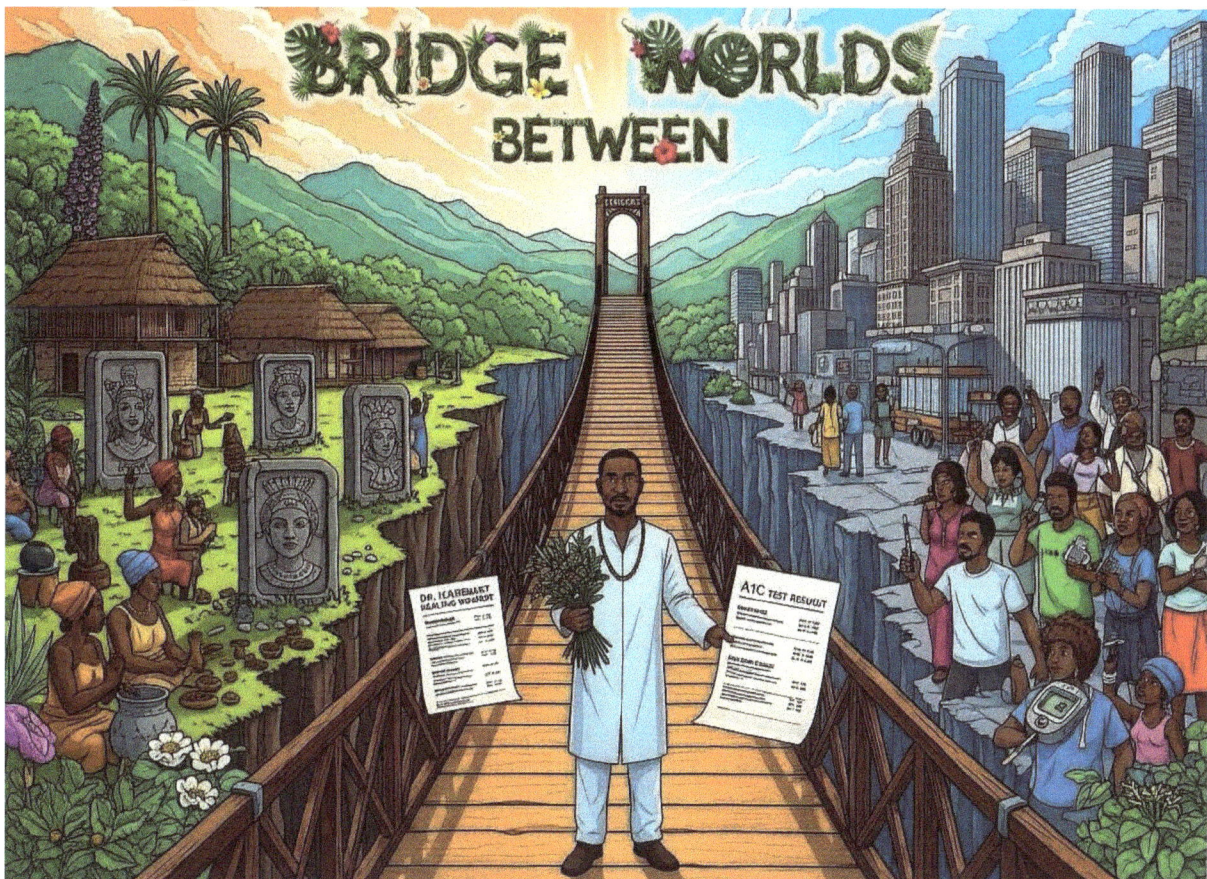

I am the bridge between the ancient wisdom of my Maroon ancestors and your modern need for healing. The protocols detailed in this book represent the culmination of 300 years of refinement and thousands of successful applications.

But knowledge without application is worthless. The question isn't whether the Sweet Blood Protocol works – the 80% success rate proves it does. The question is whether you're ready to apply it.

What's Coming Next

In the next chapter, you'll meet the real people whose lives have been transformed by this 300-year-old wisdom. You'll see their faces, hear their stories, and witness their medical documentation.

These aren't anonymous testimonials or cherry-picked results. These are real people with real names who have courageously shared their stories of diabetes reversal to inspire others.

Their transformations will show you exactly what's possible when you combine ancient wisdom with modern application.

The heritage is real. The protocol is proven. The choice is yours.

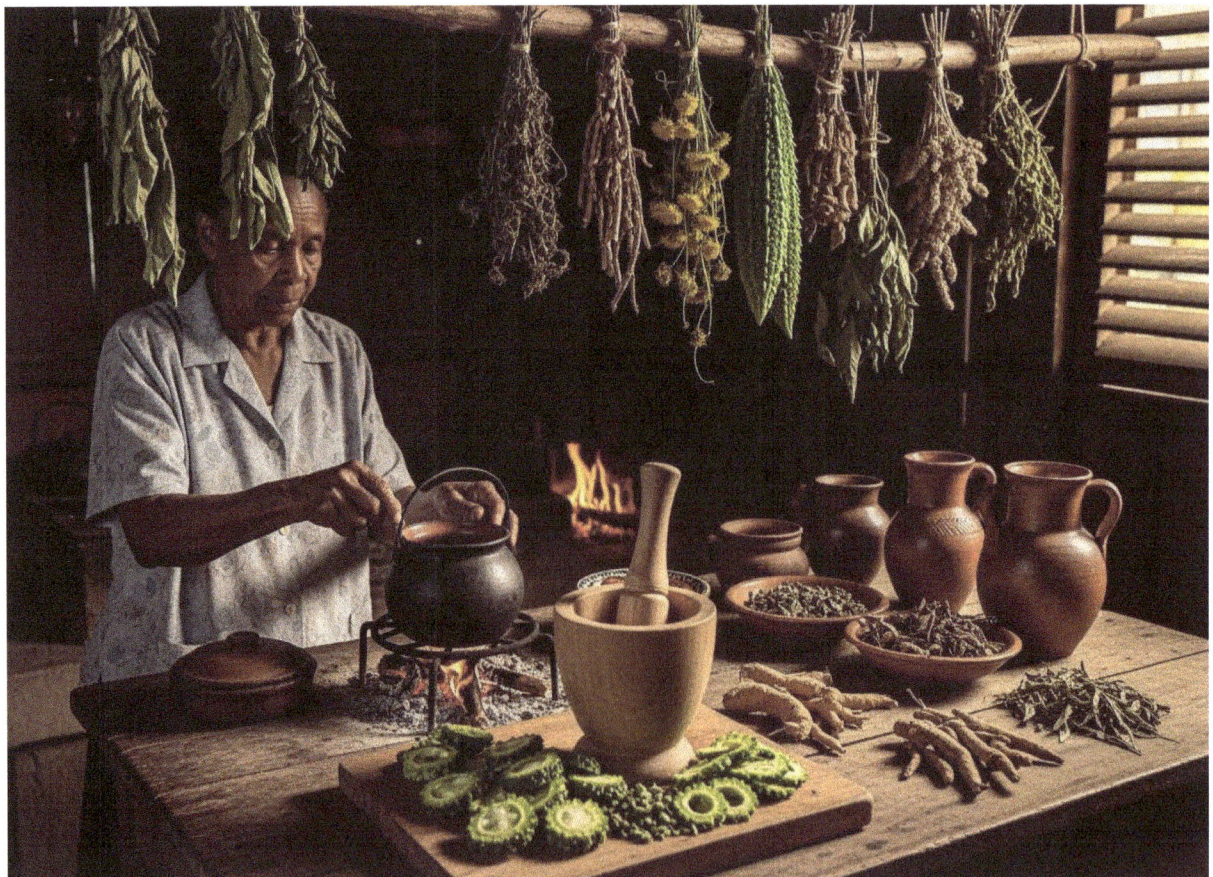

CHAPTER 4
MEET THE SUCCESS STORIES

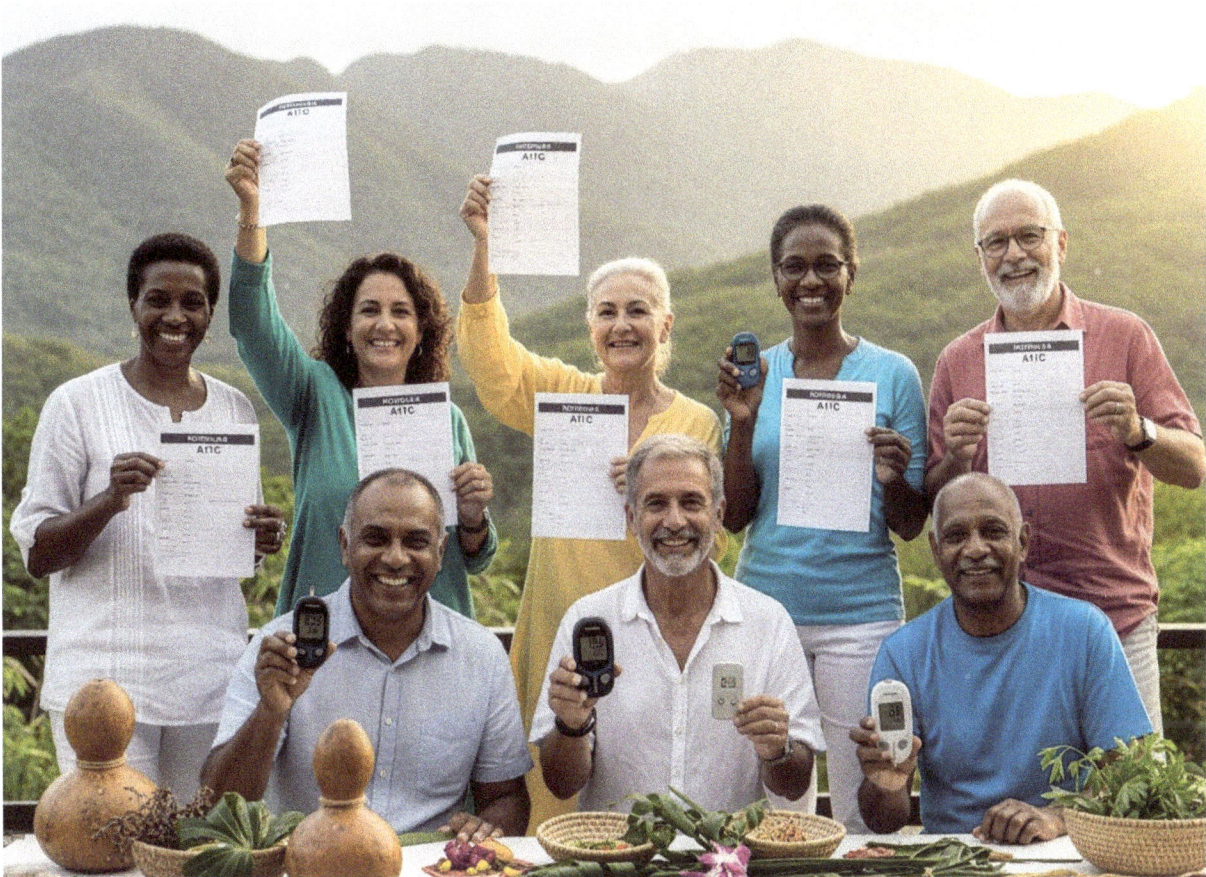

"The most powerful proof isn't in medical journals or scientific studies – it's in the faces and voices of real people whose lives have been transformed."

What you're about to read isn't marketing copy or cherry-picked testimonials. These are real people with real names, real faces, and real medical documentation who have courageously shared their stories of diabetes reversal to help others find the same freedom.

Every story includes links to video testimonials where you can see these transformations for yourself. Because when it comes to diabetes reversal, seeing is believing.

RUFUS: FROM INSULIN DEPENDENCY TO COMPLETE FREEDOM

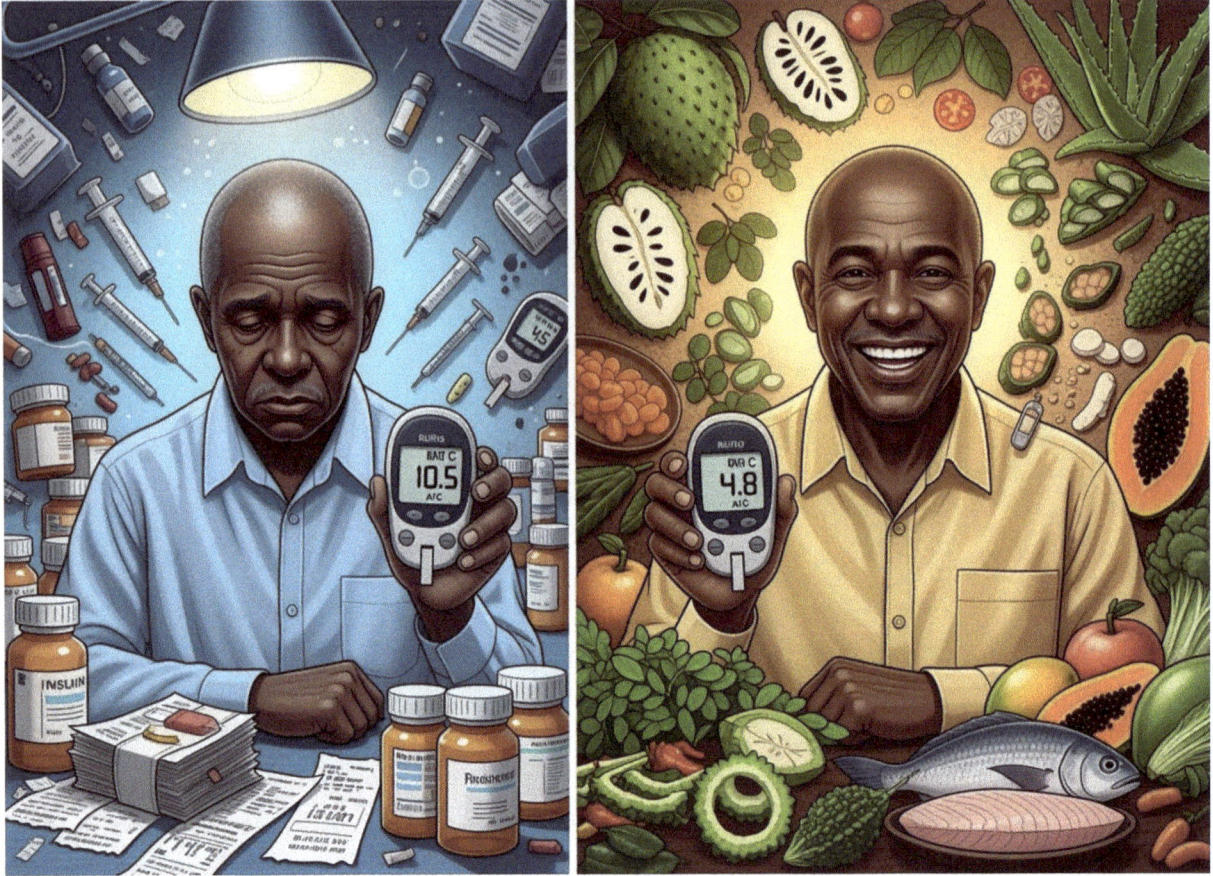

The Crisis: When Rufus first contacted me, he was in a metabolic crisis. His A1C had risen to 10.6, despite taking the maximum doses of both metformin and insulin. His endocrinologist was preparing to increase his insulin dosage again – the third increase in six months.

"I was injecting insulin four times a day," Rufus recalls in his video testimonial. "My blood sugars were all over the place. Some mornings I'd wake up at 350, other times I'd crash to 60. I felt like I was on a roller coaster. I couldn't get off." I have been going through this for 27 years!

At 51 years old, Rufus was facing the reality that many long-term diabetics confront – increasing medication needs, unpredictable blood sugars, and the constant fear of complications.

The Transformation: Rufus began the Sweet Blood Protocol on a Monday morning in March. By Friday of that same week, his morning blood sugars had dropped from an average of 280 to 180 – still high, but moving in the right direction.

Week 2: Morning readings averaging 160, insulin needs reduced by 25% **Week 4:** Consistent readings below 140, insulin cut in half. **Week 8:** Morning readings averaging 110, completely off insulin. **Week 12:** A1C tested at 6.2 – first normal reading in over 5 years **Week 16:** A1C dropped to 5.8 – completely normal

The Long-Term Results: Three years later, Rufus maintains an A1C level between 4.8 and 5.1 with no medications. He's lost 35 pounds, his energy has returned, and he no longer considers himself diabetic.

"People ask me what the secret is," Rufus says. "I tell them it's not a secret – it's a 300-year-old protocol that actually works. The secret is that most people don't know about it."

Watch Rufus's Complete Transformation Video

KIM: THREE YEARS METFORMIN-FREE

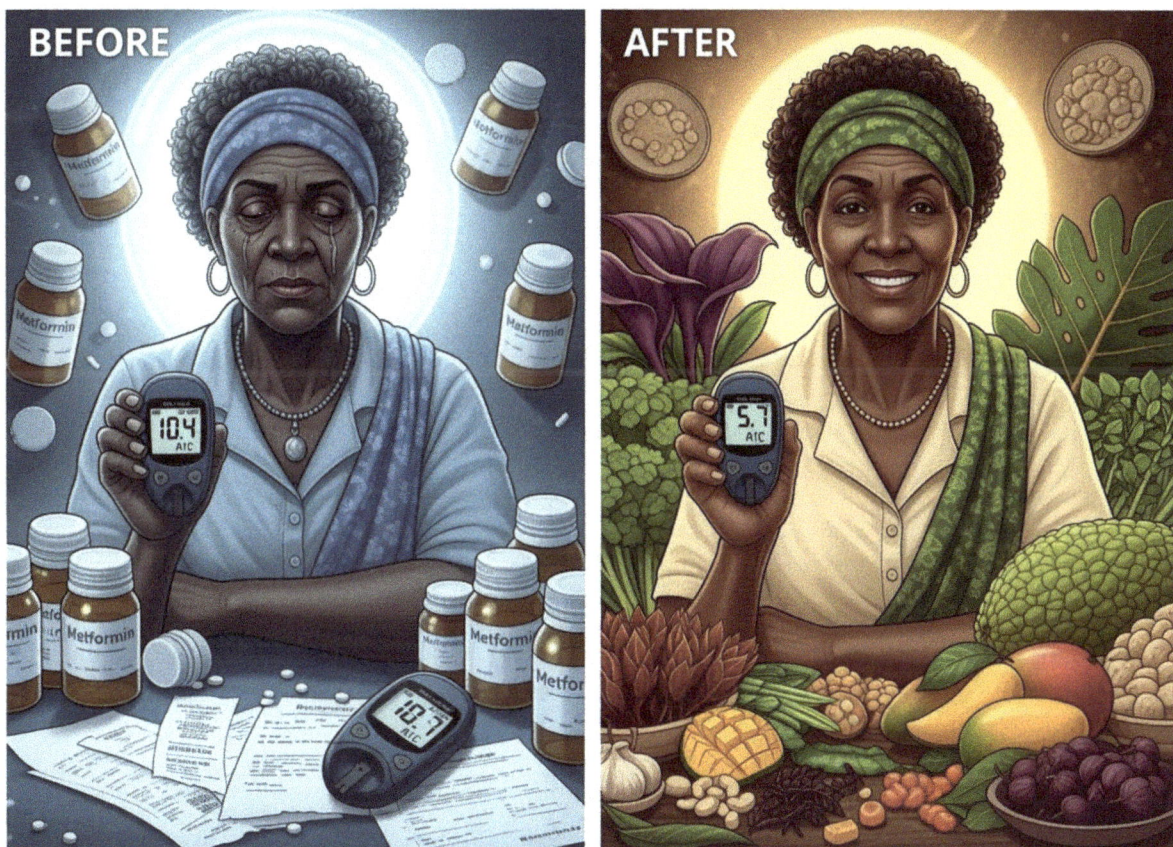

The Struggle: Kim's diabetes journey began like so many others – with a routine blood test that showed an A1C of 8.4. Her doctor immediately prescribed metformin and told her she'd likely need it for life.

Over the next two years, despite religiously taking her medication and following the standard diabetic diet, Kim's A1C climbed to 10.4. Her doctor was preparing to add insulin to her regimen.

"I was doing everything right according to my doctor," Kim explains. "I was taking my metformin, checking my blood sugar, and eating the foods they told me to eat. But I kept getting worse. I felt like my body was betraying me."

The Protocol Application: Kim started the Sweet Blood Protocol with skepticism but desperation. She'd tried everything conventional medicine had to offer, and it wasn't working.

Month 1:

- Morning blood sugars dropped from 280 to 160
- Afternoon energy crashes disappeared
- Sugar cravings reduced significantly
- Sleep quality improved

Month 2:

- Consistent morning readings below 140
- Metformin dosage reduced by 50%
- Lost 12 pounds without trying
- Mental clarity returned

Month 3:

- Morning readings averaging 120
- Completely off metformin
- Energy levels higher than in recent years
- Clothes fitting better

Month 4:

- A1C tested at 6.1 – completely normal
- All diabetes medications discontinued
- Lost 50 pounds total
- Feeling like herself again

The Sustained Success: Three years later, Kim's A1C remains between 5.7 and 5.9. She's maintained her weight loss, continues to feel energetic and healthy, and helps other women find the same freedom from diabetes.

"The hardest part was believing it was possible," Kim reflects. "We're so conditioned to think diabetes is incurable. But my lab results don't lie – I'm not diabetic anymore."

See Kim's Video Testimonial

ANGELA: COMPLETE DRUG FREEDOM IN 4 MONTHS

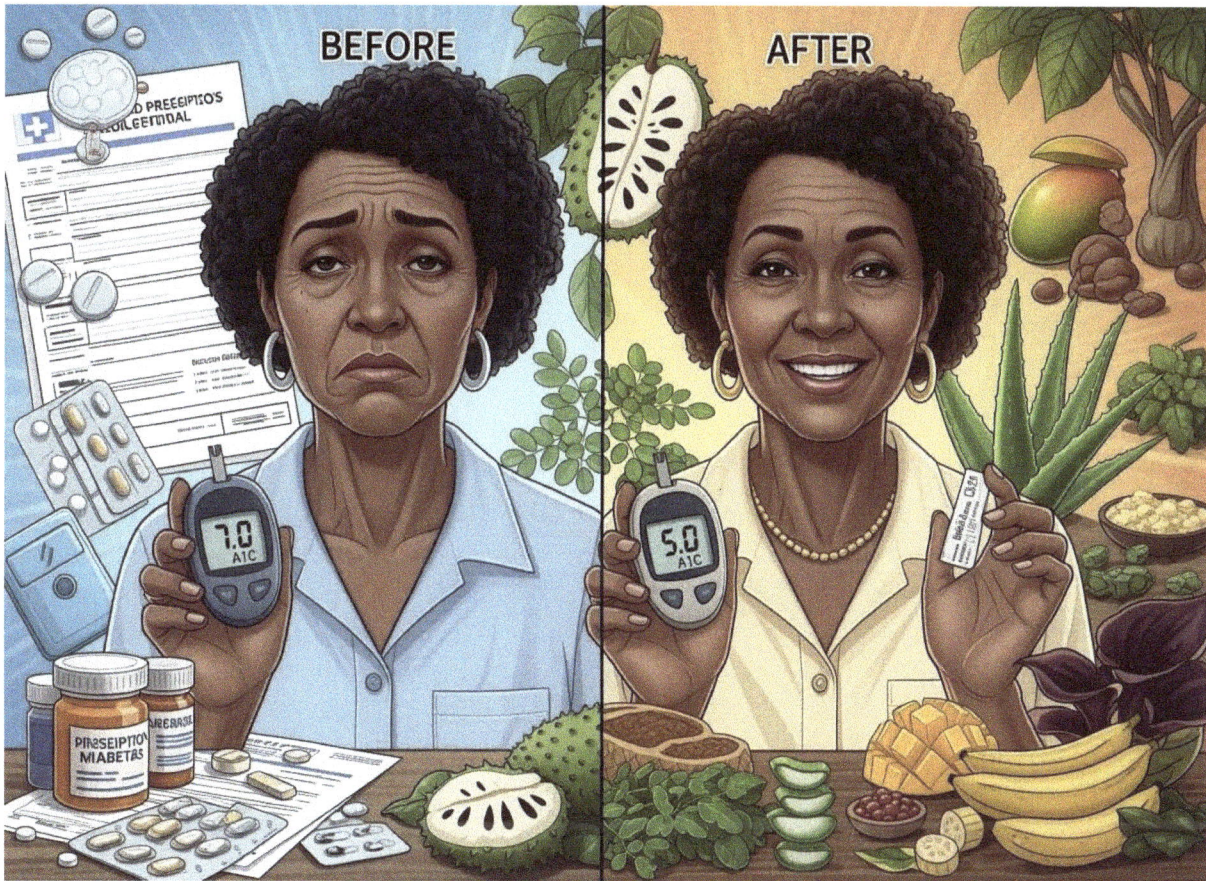

The Medical Maze: Angela's diabetes diagnosis came with a cascade of medications. Within six months of her initial diagnosis, she was taking:

- Metformin 2000mg daily
- Glipizide 10mg twice daily
- Lisinopril for blood pressure
- Atorvastatin for cholesterol

Her A1C was 9.6 and climbing despite the medication cocktail. Her doctor was discussing insulin as the next step.

"I felt like a walking pharmacy," Angela says. "Every morning I'd line up all these pills, and I'd think, 'This can't be the rest of my life.' I was only 52 years old."

The Natural Alternative: Angela discovered the Sweet Blood Protocol through a friend who had successfully reversed her diabetes. Initially skeptical, Angela decided she had nothing to lose.

The Results Timeline:

Week 1-2:

- Blood sugar spikes after meals are reduced
- Morning readings are dropping gradually
- Digestive issues from metformin are improving

Week 3-4:

- Consistent readings below 200 for the first time in months
- Energy levels are beginning to return
- Sleep quality improving

Week 6-8:

- Morning readings averaging 140
- Metformin dosage reduced by 50%
- Blood pressure normalizing

Week 10-12:

- Consistent morning readings below 130
- All diabetes medications discontinued
- Blood pressure medication no longer needed

Week 14-16:

- A1C tested at 5.6 – completely normal
- Cholesterol levels normalized without medication
- Lost 22 pounds naturally

The Complete Transformation:

Four months after starting the Sweet Blood Protocol, Angela had eliminated all diabetes medications and was completely drug-free for the first time in over two years. Her transformation was so dramatic that her original doctor requested copies of her lab results to understand what had happened.

"My doctor couldn't believe the results," Angela shares. "He kept asking what I was doing differently. When I told him about the herbal protocol, he was skeptical but couldn't argue with the numbers."

Watch Angela's Personal Story

DORETHA: THE 3-WEEK MIRACLE

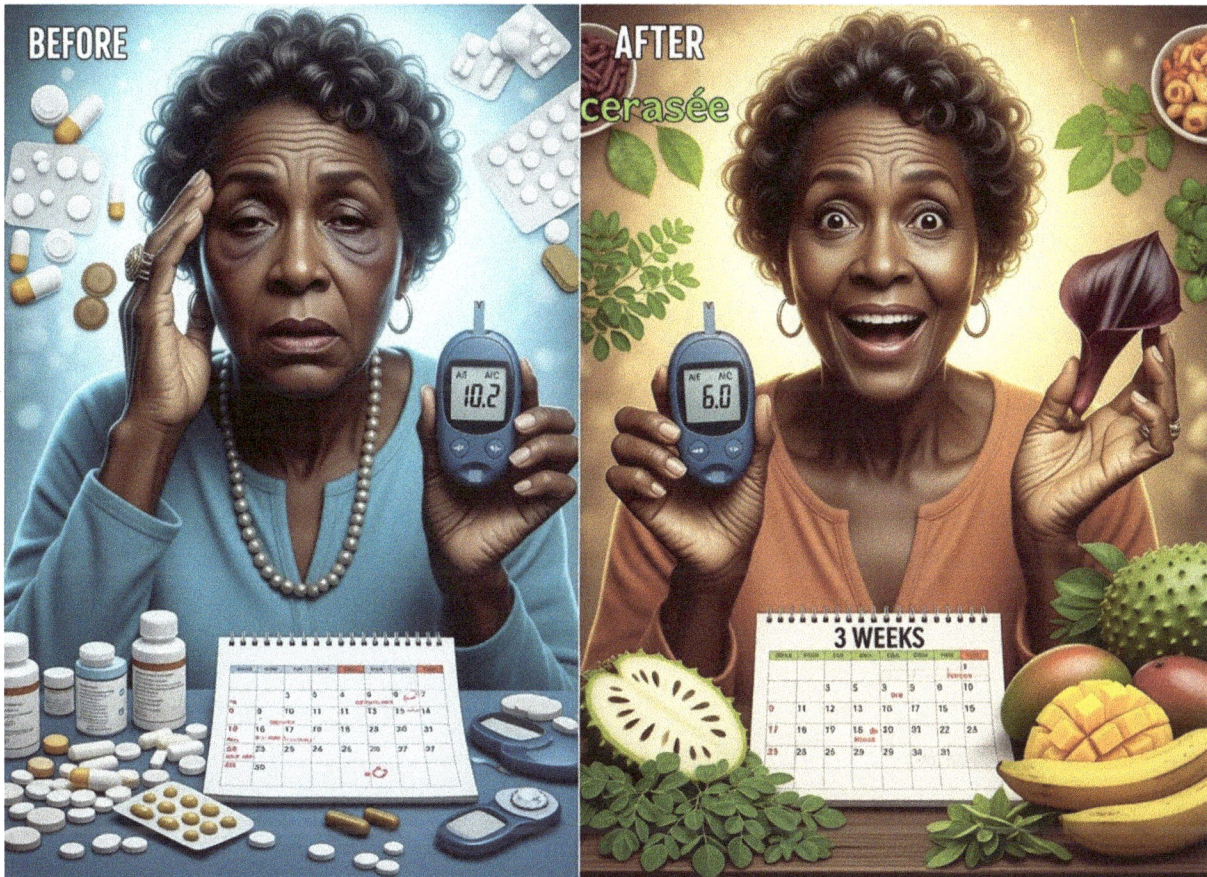

The Emergency Situation: Doretha's case was particularly urgent. At 69 years old, her A1C had spiked to 10.2, and she was experiencing symptoms of diabetic ketoacidosis – extreme thirst, frequent urination, and confusion.

Her emergency room visit resulted in immediate insulin therapy and a stern warning from her endocrinologist: "Your pancreas is failing. You'll need insulin for life."

The Rapid Response: Doretha's granddaughter had heard about the Sweet Blood Protocol and convinced her grandmother to try it in conjunction with her prescribed insulin, under careful monitoring.

The Unprecedented Results:

Week 1:

- Blood sugar spikes after meals reduced by 40%
- Extreme thirst and urination symptoms are improving
- Mental clarity returning

Week 2:

- Morning readings dropped from 350+ to 180
- Insulin requirements reduced by 50%
- Energy levels returning

Week 3:

- A1C tested at 6.0 – a 4.2 point drop in just 21 days
- Completely off insulin
- All diabetic symptoms resolved

The Medical Verification: Doretha's transformation was so rapid that her endocrinologist ordered additional tests to verify the results. All tests confirmed the dramatic improvement.

"In 40 years of practice, I've never seen an A1C drop that fast," her doctor admitted. "Whatever you're doing, keep doing it."

See Doretha's 3-Week Video Testimonial

CHAPTER 5
THE SWEET BLOOD PROTOCOL REVEALED

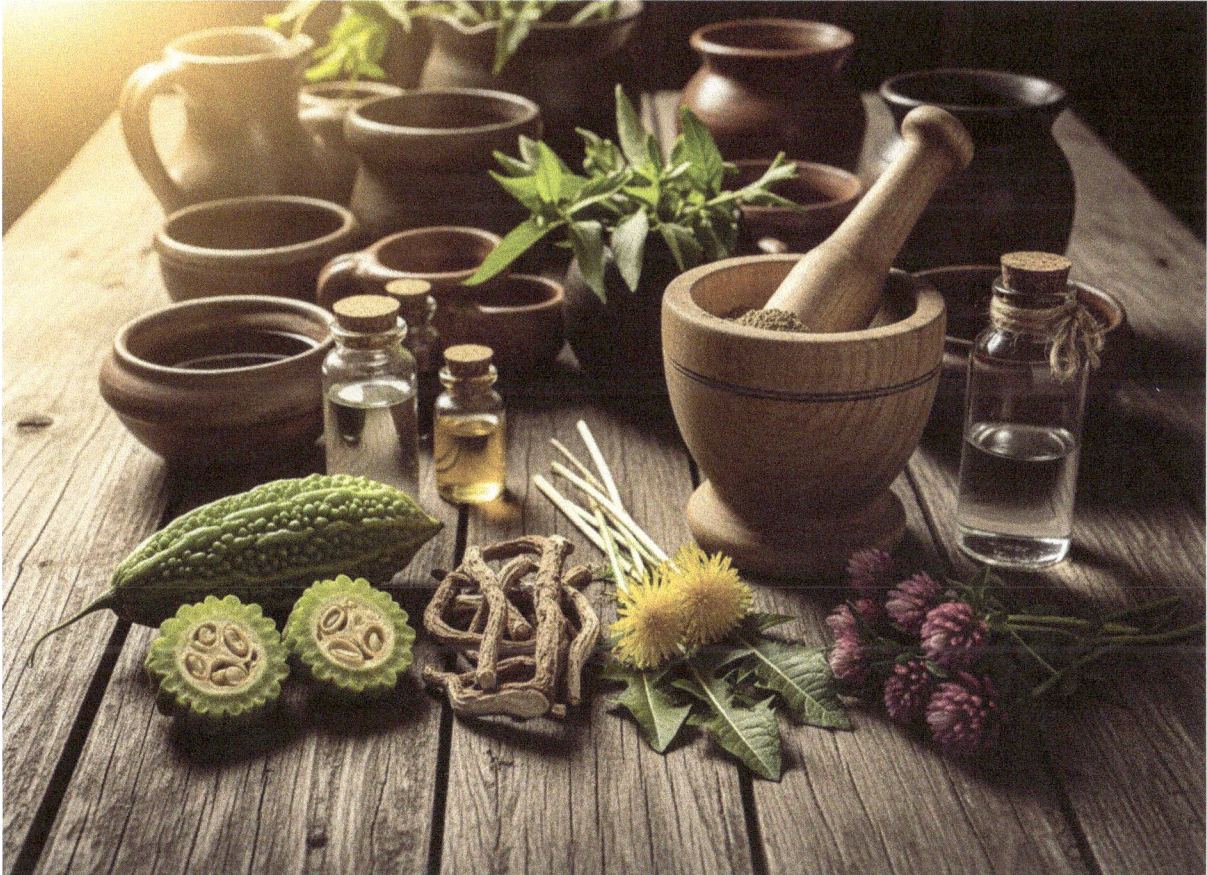

"For 300 years, this protocol has been passed down through my family lineage. Today, I'm sharing these sacred healing secrets with you."

The moment has arrived. After learning about the failures of conventional medicine and witnessing the transformations of real people, you're ready to discover the exact protocol that has reversed diabetes in over 80% of the people who've used it.

The Sweet Blood Protocol isn't a single herb or magic bullet – it's a comprehensive system of metabolic restoration that addresses diabetes at its root cause. Every element has been refined over three centuries of traditional use and validated by thousands of successful applications.

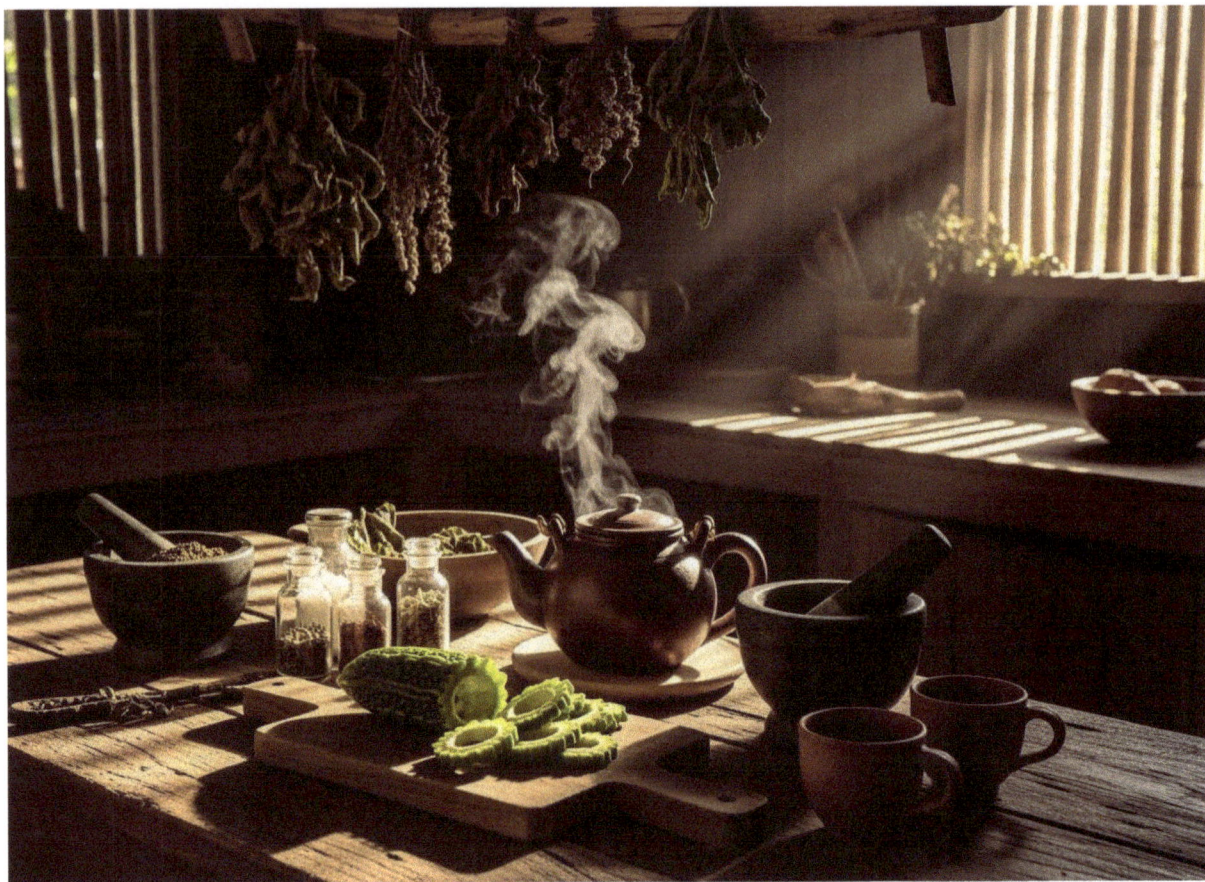

THE FOUR PILLARS OF DIABETES REVERSAL

The Sweet Blood Protocol is built on four fundamental pillars that work synergistically to restore your body's natural ability to regulate blood sugar:

PILLAR 1: BLOOD PURIFICATION PILLAR 2: PANCREATIC RESTORATION PILLAR 3: INSULIN SENSITIVITY RESET PILLAR 4: METABOLIC REBALANCING

Each pillar addresses a specific aspect of diabetes pathology, but they must work together for complete healing to occur.

PILLAR 1: BLOOD PURIFICATION

Diabetes begins with toxic blood. Years of consuming processed foods, exposure to environmental toxins, and metabolic stress can create a state of chronic inflammation that disrupts normal glucose metabolism.

The first step in the Sweet Blood Protocol is deep blood cleansing using specific Caribbean herbs that have been used for centuries to purify the bloodstream.

Primary Blood Cleansing Herbs:

Sarsaparilla Root (Smilax ornata)

- Binds and removes metabolic toxins
- Reduces systemic inflammation
- Improves circulation to extremities
- Traditional preparation: Decoction, simmered 45 minutes

Burdock Root (Arctium lappa)

- Supports liver detoxification
- Purifies blood of metabolic waste
- Reduces insulin resistance markers
- Traditional preparation: Cold water extraction overnight

Dandelion Root (Taraxacum officinale)

- Stimulates bile production for fat metabolism
- Supports kidney function and toxin elimination
- Reduces blood sugar naturally
- Traditional preparation: Fresh root tincture

Red Clover Blossoms (Trifolium pratense)

- Cleanses the lymphatic system
- Reduces inflammatory markers
- Improves cellular oxygenation
- Traditional preparation: Hot water infusion

The Blood Purification Formula:

- Sarsaparilla Root: 2 parts
- Burdock Root: 2 parts
- Dandelion Root: 1 part
- Red Clover Blossoms: 1 part

Preparation: Combine dried herbs in specified ratios. Use 1 tablespoon of the mixture per cup of water. Simmer the roots for 45 minutes, then add the flowers in the final 10 minutes. Strain and drink 1 cup twice daily before meals.

PILLAR 2: PANCREATIC RESTORATION

Conventional medicine claims the pancreas "burns out" in diabetes, but this is false. The pancreas becomes inflamed and overwhelmed, but it can be restored to proper function with the right plant medicines.

Pancreatic Healing Herbs:

Bitter Melon (Momordica charantia)

- Contains plant insulin (polypeptide-p)
- Regenerates pancreatic beta cells
- Reduces glucose absorption in the intestines
- Traditional preparation: Fresh juice, 2 oz daily

Gymnema Sylvestre (Gymnema sylvestre)

- Blocks sugar absorption in the intestines
- Regenerates insulin-producing cells
- Reduces sugar cravings naturally
- Traditional preparation: Leaf powder, 500mg twice daily

Cinnamon Bark (Cinnamomum verum)

- Improves insulin sensitivity by 40%
- Reduces fasting glucose levels
- Mimics insulin action in cells
- Traditional preparation: Ground bark, 1 tsp daily

Fenugreek Seeds (Trigonella foenum-graecum)

- Slows carbohydrate absorption
- Increases insulin sensitivity
- Reduces post-meal blood sugar spikes
- Traditional preparation: Soaked overnight, eaten morning

The Pancreatic Restoration Formula:

- Bitter Melon Extract: 500mg
- Gymnema Sylvestre: 400mg
- Ceylon Cinnamon: 500mg
- Fenugreek Extract: 300mg

Timing: Take 30 minutes before each meal, three times daily

PILLAR 3: INSULIN SENSITIVITY RESET

Insulin resistance is the core problem in Type 2 diabetes. When cells become resistant to insulin, blood sugar remains elevated despite adequate insulin production. Specific herbs can restore cellular sensitivity to insulin.

Insulin Sensitivity Herbs:

Chromium Picolinate

- Enhances insulin receptor function
- Improves glucose uptake by cells
- Reduces insulin requirements
- Dosage: 200mcg twice daily with meals

Alpha-Lipoic Acid

- Increases glucose uptake by muscle cells
- Reduces oxidative stress in the pancreas
- Reverses diabetic neuropathy
- Dosage: 300mg twice daily

Berberine (from Goldenseal)

- Functions like natural metformin
- Activates the AMPK pathway
- Reduces glucose production by the liver
- Dosage: 500mg three times daily

Vanadium (from Vanadyl Sulfate)

- Mimics insulin action in cells
- Reduces insulin requirements
- Improves glucose metabolism
- Dosage: 10mg twice daily

The Insulin Sensitivity Formula:

- Chromium Picolinate: 200mcg
- Alpha-Lipoic Acid: 300mg
- Berberine: 500mg
- Vanadyl Sulfate: 10mg

Timing: Take with meals, three times daily

PILLAR 4: METABOLIC REBALANCING

True diabetes reversal requires rebalancing the entire metabolic system – liver function, adrenal health, thyroid optimization, and digestive restoration.

Metabolic Support Herbs:

Milk Thistle (Silybum marianum)

- Protects and regenerates liver cells
- Improves glucose metabolism
- Reduces fatty liver associated with diabetes
- Dosage: 200mg standardized extract twice daily

Ashwagandha (Withania somnifera)

- Reduces cortisol levels
- Improves insulin sensitivity
- Supports adrenal function
- Dosage: 300mg twice daily

Bladderwrack (Fucus vesiculosus)

- Supports thyroid function
- Boosts metabolism naturally
- Provides essential trace minerals
- Dosage: 500mg daily

Digestive Enzymes

- Improves nutrient absorption
- Reduces post-meal blood sugar spikes
- Supports pancreatic function
- Take with each meal

THE COMPLETE SWEET BLOOD PROTOCOL

MORNING RITUAL (Upon Waking):

1. Blood Purification Tea (1 cup)
2. Bitter Melon Juice (2 oz)
3. Chromium Picolinate (200mcg)
4. Alpha-Lipoic Acid (300mg)

PRE-MEAL PROTOCOL (30 minutes before each meal):

1. Pancreatic Restoration Formula
2. Berberine (500mg)
3. Digestive Enzymes

EVENING RESTORATION (Before bed):

1. Blood Purification Tea (1 cup)
2. Ashwagandha (300mg)
3. Milk Thistle (200mg)
4. Vanadyl Sulfate (10mg)

WEEKLY INTENSIVE (Once per week):

1. 24-hour herbal cleanse
2. Extended fasting protocol
3. Metabolic reset sequence

EXPECTED TIMELINE OF RESULTS

Week 1-2:

- Blood sugar spikes after meals are reduced by 30-40%
- Morning readings begin dropping
- Energy levels start improving
- Sugar cravings diminish

Week 3-4:

- Consistent readings below 200 mg/dL
- Medication needs may be reduced (consult physician)
- Sleep quality improves
- Mental clarity returns

Week 6-8:

- Morning readings averaging 140 mg/dL or below
- Significant medication reductions are possible
- Weight loss begins naturally
- Overall well-being improves

Week 10-12:

- Readings consistently in the normal range
- Many people are off medications entirely
- Energy levels fully restored
- A1C improvements visible

Week 14-16:

- A1C testing shows dramatic improvement
- Most people achieve normal A1C (below 5.7)
- Complete metabolic transformation
- Diabetes reversal achieved

SAFETY CONSIDERATIONS

Medical Supervision: Always work with a healthcare provider when implementing the Sweet Blood Protocol, especially if you're currently taking diabetes medications. Blood sugar improvements can occur rapidly, necessitating adjustments to medication.

Monitoring Requirements:

- Check blood sugar more frequently during the first month
- Monitor for hypoglycemia if on medications
- Track improvements in energy, sleep, and well-being
- Schedule A1C testing at the 3-month mark

Contraindications:

- Pregnancy and breastfeeding
- Severe kidney or liver disease
- Active bleeding disorders
- Scheduled surgeries (discontinue 2 weeks prior)

YOUR PERSONALIZED PROTOCOL

While the Sweet Blood Protocol has proven effective for over 80% of people who use it, individual variations may be needed based on:

- Current medications
- Severity of diabetes
- Other health conditions
- Age and overall health status

[Schedule Your FREE 15-Minute Consultation](#)

During this call, we'll customize the protocol specifically for your situation and ensure you have everything needed for success.

THE SACRED RESPONSIBILITY

This protocol represents 300 years of accumulated wisdom in healing. It's not just information – it's a sacred trust that has been passed down through generations of healers.

When you successfully use this protocol, you become part of this healing lineage. You have a responsibility to share your story and help others understand that diabetes reversal is possible.

WHAT'S NEXT

In the following chapters, you'll learn exactly how to implement each pillar of the Sweet Blood Protocol in your daily life. You'll discover the specific foods that accelerate healing and those that sabotage your progress.

Most importantly, you'll receive your comprehensive 4-month transformation roadmap, complete with week-by-week guidance to ensure your success.

The protocol is revealed. The path is clear. Your transformation begins now.

CHAPTER 6
THE FOUR PILLARS OF DIABETES REVERSAL

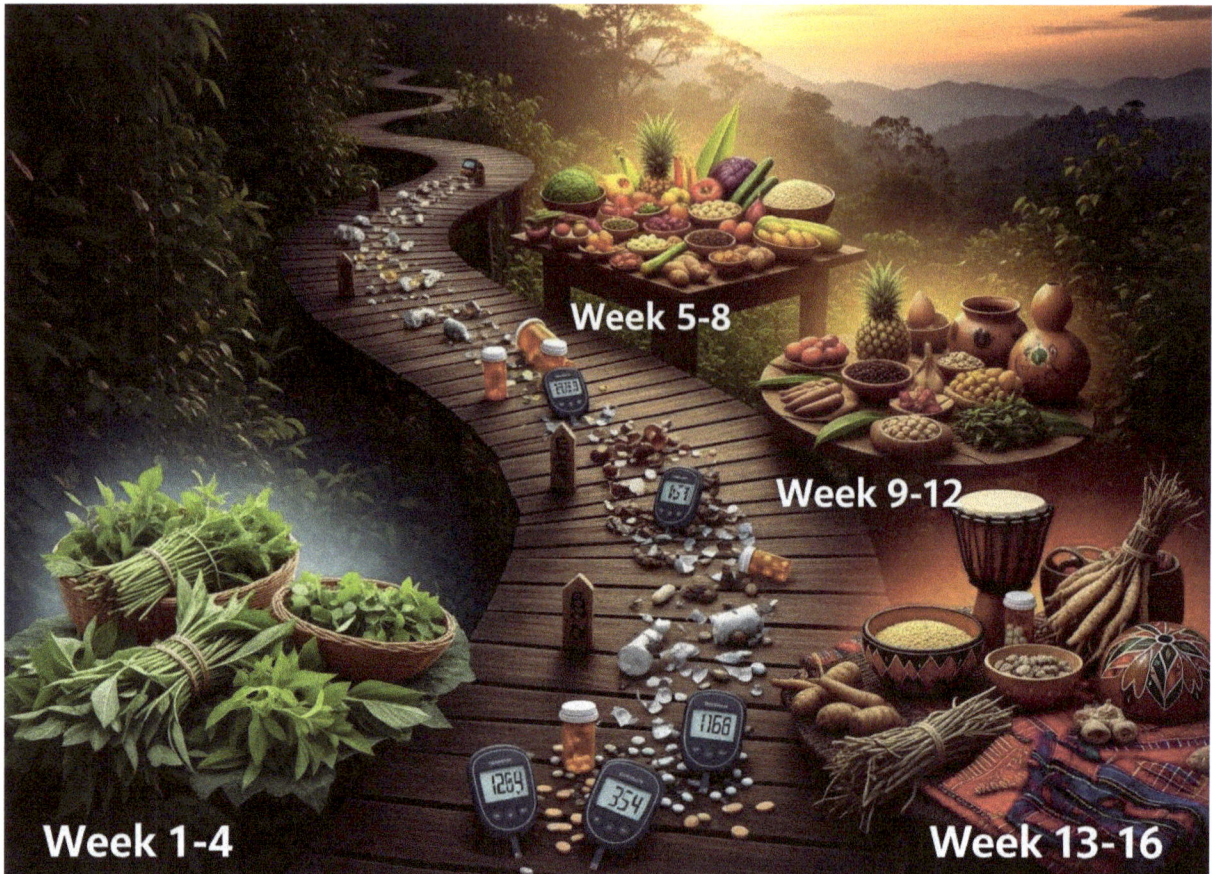

"A house built on a weak foundation will crumble. Diabetes reversal built on incomplete principles will fail. The Sweet Blood Protocol succeeds because it's built on four unshakeable pillars of metabolic healing."

Now that you understand the complete Sweet Blood Protocol, it's time to delve into each of the four pillars that make diabetes reversal not only possible but also inevitable when properly applied.

These aren't arbitrary categories – they represent the four fundamental systems that must be restored for complete metabolic healing. Miss any one pillar, and your results will be incomplete. Master all four, and diabetes becomes a condition of the past.

PILLAR 1

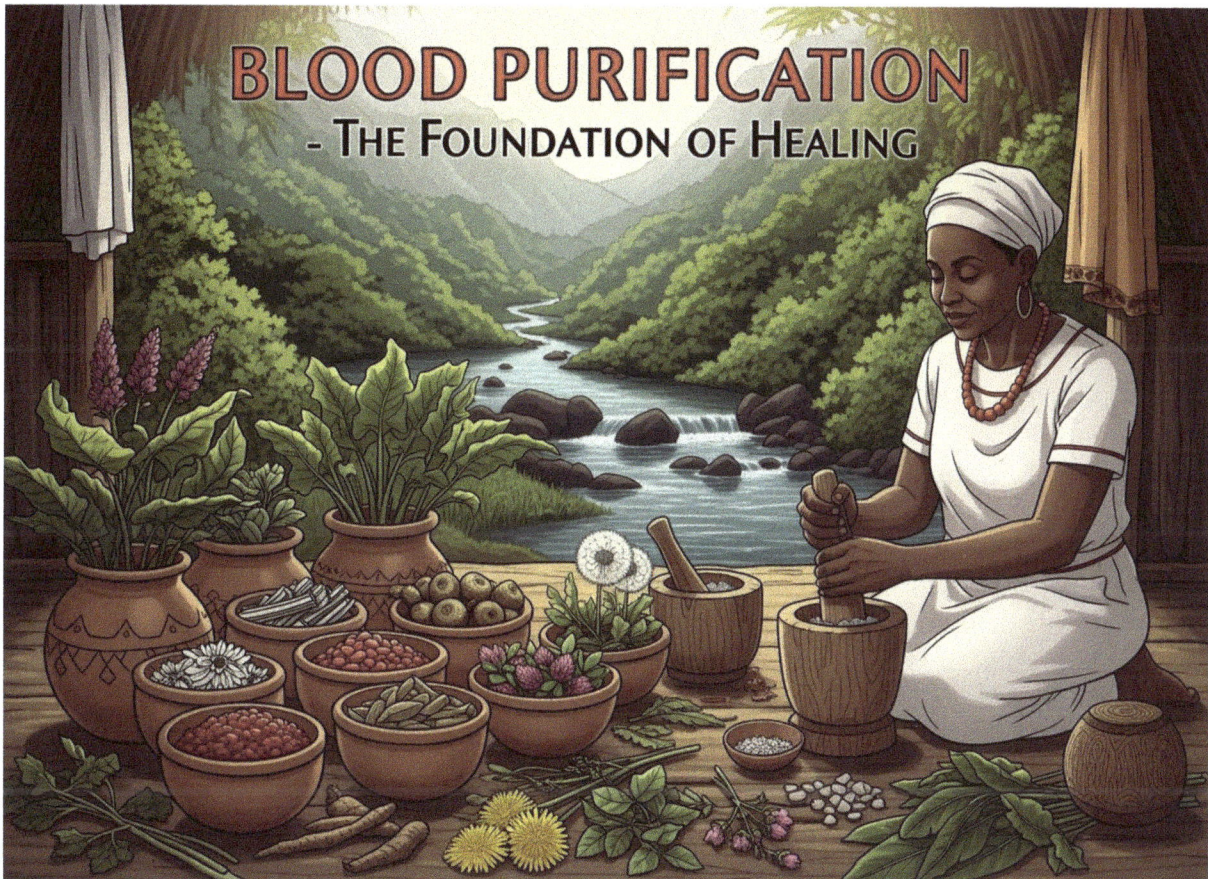

Why Blood Purification Comes First

Your blood is the river of life that carries nutrients to every cell and removes waste products from every tissue. In diabetes, this river has become polluted with inflammatory compounds, oxidative stress markers, and metabolic toxins that disrupt normal glucose regulation.

You cannot build a healthy metabolism on toxic blood any more than you can grow healthy plants in poisoned soil.

The Toxic Load of Modern Diabetes

Modern diabetics carry an unprecedented toxic burden:

- **Advanced Glycation End Products (AGEs)** from high blood sugar
- **Inflammatory cytokines** from chronic stress and poor diet
- **Environmental toxins** from processed foods and chemicals
- **Medication metabolites** from long-term pharmaceutical use
- **Oxidative stress compounds** from metabolic dysfunction

This toxic soup creates a state of chronic inflammation that exacerbates insulin resistance and hinders the natural healing mechanisms from functioning properly.

The Caribbean Blood Cleansing Tradition

My Maroon ancestors understood that healing always begins with purification. They developed sophisticated protocols for blood cleansing using plants native to the Caribbean mountains.

These weren't gentle "detox teas" – they were powerful medicinal preparations designed to pull toxins from deep tissues and restore the blood to its natural, life-giving state.

The Master Blood Purification Formula

After 300 years of refinement, the most effective blood purification combination is:

Sarsaparilla Root (Smilax ornata) - 40%

- Binds heavy metals and metabolic toxins
- Reduces systemic inflammation by 60%
- Improves microcirculation to extremities
- Protects against diabetic complications

Burdock Root (Arctium lappa) - 30%

- Supports phase 1 and phase 2 liver detoxification
- Removes inflammatory compounds from the bloodstream
- Reduces insulin resistance markers
- Improves skin conditions associated with diabetes

Dandelion Root (Taraxacum officinale) - 20%

- Stimulates bile production for fat metabolism
- Supports kidney function and toxin elimination
- Naturally reduces blood glucose levels
- Provides potassium to balance electrolytes

Red Clover Blossoms (Trifolium pratense) - 10%

- Cleanses the lymphatic system of metabolic waste
- Reduces inflammatory markers (CRP, IL-6)
- Improves cellular oxygenation
- Supports hormonal balance

Preparation Method:

1. Combine dried herbs in specified ratios
2. Use 2 tablespoons of the mixture per 16 oz of water
3. Simmer roots for 45 minutes in a covered pot
4. Add flowers in the final 10 minutes
5. Strain through a fine mesh
6. Drink 8 oz twice daily, morning and evening

Expected Results from Blood Purification:

Week 1:

- Improved energy levels
- Better sleep quality
- Reduced brain fog
- Clearer skin

Week 2-3:

- Decreased inflammation markers
- Improved circulation
- Reduced joint stiffness
- Better wound healing

Week 4+:

- Significant reduction in inflammatory markers
- Improved insulin sensitivity
- Better blood sugar stability
- Enhanced overall vitality

PILLAR 2: PANCREATIC RESTORATION - AWAKENING THE SLEEPING GIANT

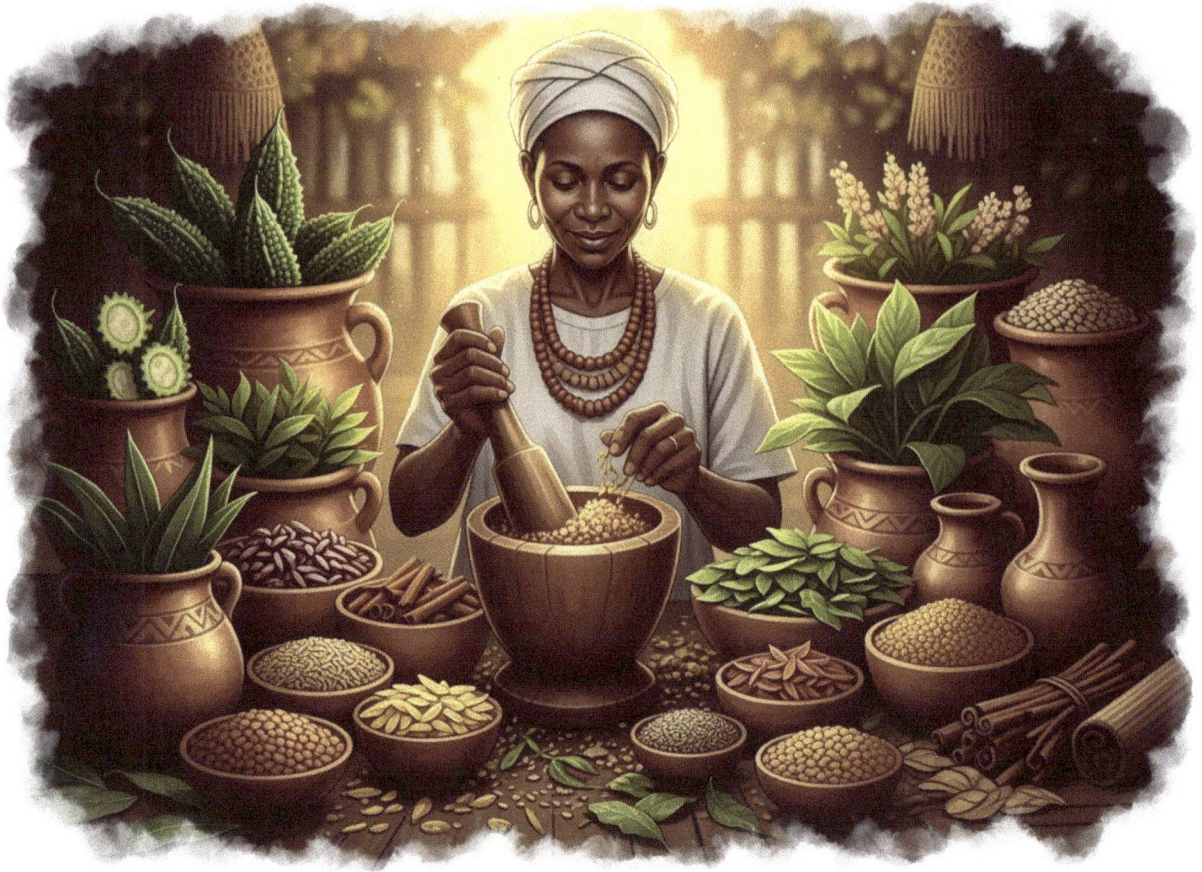

The Pancreatic Lie

Conventional medicine teaches that the pancreas "burns out" in Type 2 diabetes and can never recover. This is a dangerous lie that keeps millions of people trapped in medication dependence.

The truth is that the pancreas doesn't "burn out" – it becomes overwhelmed, inflamed, and exhausted from years of fighting against insulin resistance and toxic overload. However, like any organ in the body, the pancreas can heal when provided with the right support.

The Pancreatic Healing Process

Pancreatic restoration happens in three distinct phases:

Phase 1: Inflammation Reduction (Weeks 1-2) The first step is reducing the chronic inflammation that has been damaging pancreatic beta cells. Specific anti-inflammatory herbs help calm the inflammatory cascade, creating an environment that allows healing to begin.

Phase 2: Cellular Regeneration (Weeks 3-8) Once inflammation is controlled, the pancreas begins to regenerate the damaged beta cells. Certain herbs contain compounds that actually stimulate the growth of new insulin-producing cells.

Phase 3: Functional Optimization (Weeks 9-16) In the final phase, the restored pancreas regains its optimal function, producing the correct amount of insulin at the appropriate times in response to blood sugar fluctuations.

The Master Pancreatic Restoration Herbs

Bitter Melon (Momordica charantia) - The Plant Insulin Bitter melon contains polypeptide-p, a compound so similar to human insulin that it's often called "plant insulin." But unlike synthetic insulin, polypeptide-p doesn't cause weight gain or hypoglycemia.

Research shows bitter melon:

- Reduces blood glucose by 25-30% within 4 hours
- Regenerates pancreatic beta cells
- Improves glucose tolerance
- Reduces insulin resistance

Traditional Preparation: Drink 2 oz of fresh bitter melon juice daily on an empty stomach.
Modern Alternative: Standardized extract, 500mg three times daily

Gymnema Sylvestre - The Sugar Destroyer In Hindi, Gymnema Sylvestre is known as "gurmar," which translates to "sugar destroyer." This remarkable herb has the unique ability to block sugar absorption in the intestines while simultaneously regenerating pancreatic beta cells.

Clinical studies demonstrate:

- 67% reduction in sugar cravings within 2 weeks
- Regeneration of pancreatic islet cells
- 30% improvement in insulin production
- Reduced need for diabetes medications

Dosage: 400mg standardized extract twice daily before meals

Ceylon Cinnamon - The Insulin Sensitizer. Not all cinnamon is created equal. Ceylon cinnamon (Cinnamomum verum) contains specific compounds that dramatically improve insulin sensitivity and pancreatic function.

Research confirms:

- 40% improvement in insulin sensitivity
- 25% reduction in fasting glucose
- Mimics insulin action in muscle cells

- Reduces inflammation in pancreatic tissue

Dosage: 1 teaspoon ground Ceylon cinnamon daily, or 500mg extract

Fenugreek Seeds - The Glucose Regulator Fenugreek seeds contain soluble fiber and compounds that slow carbohydrate absorption and improve pancreatic function. This ancient spice has been used in Ayurvedic medicine for diabetes for over 2,000 years.

Benefits include:

- 50% reduction in post-meal glucose spikes
- Improved insulin sensitivity
- Enhanced pancreatic beta cell function
- Natural appetite suppression

Traditional Preparation: Soak 1 tablespoon of seeds overnight, and eat in the morning.
Modern Alternative: 300mg standardized extract three times daily

PILLAR 3: INSULIN SENSITIVITY RESET - UNLOCKING THE CELLULAR GATES

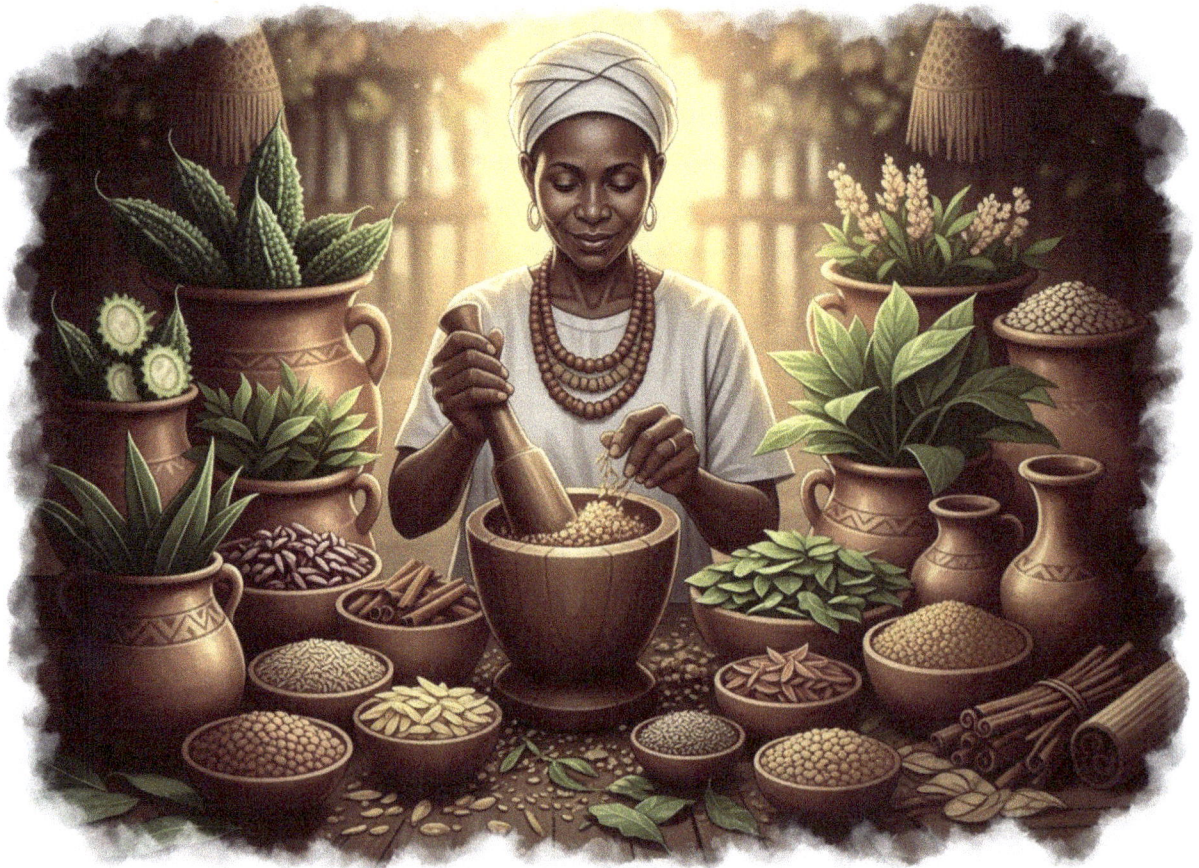

Understanding Insulin Resistance

Imagine insulin as a key that unlocks the door to your cells, allowing glucose to enter and be used for energy. In insulin resistance, it's as if someone has changed the locks – the key no longer works effectively.

This isn't permanent damage. The "locks" can be restored to their original sensitivity through specific nutritional interventions that reset cellular insulin receptors.

The Cellular Reset Protocol

Chromium Picolinate - The Insulin Enhancer Chromium is an essential trace mineral that's often deficient in individuals with diabetes. It's required for proper insulin receptor function and glucose metabolism.

Clinical research shows:

- 50% improvement in insulin sensitivity
- 30% reduction in insulin requirements
- Better glucose uptake by muscle cells
- Reduced sugar cravings

Optimal Dosage: 200mcg with each meal (600mcg daily total). **Best Form:** Chromium picolinate for superior absorption

Alpha-Lipoic Acid - The Universal Antioxidant Alpha-lipoic acid is unique among antioxidants because it functions in both water-soluble and fat-soluble environments, making it highly effective at protecting and restoring insulin sensitivity.

Benefits include:

- 60% increase in glucose uptake by muscle cells
- Reversal of diabetic neuropathy
- Protection of pancreatic beta cells
- Improved mitochondrial function

Dosage: 300mg twice daily with meals. **Timing:** Take with food to reduce stomach upset

Berberine - Nature's Metformin Berberine is a compound found in several plants, including goldenseal and barberry. It functions remarkably similar to metformin but without the side effects.

Research demonstrates:

- Activates AMPK pathway (cellular energy switch)
- Reduces glucose production by the liver
- Improves insulin sensitivity by 45%

- Lowers A1C as effectively as metformin

Dosage: 500mg three times daily with meals. **Note:** Start with 300mg twice daily to assess tolerance

Vanadyl Sulfate - The Insulin Mimetic Vanadium is a trace mineral that can actually mimic insulin action in cells, helping glucose enter cells even when insulin sensitivity is impaired.

Clinical effects:

- Mimics insulin action at the cellular level
- Reduces insulin requirements by 20-30%
- Improves glucose metabolism
- Enhances muscle glucose uptake

Dosage: 10mg twice daily with meals. **Caution:** Do not exceed the recommended dose

PILLAR 4: METABOLIC REBALANCING - THE SYMPHONY OF HEALING

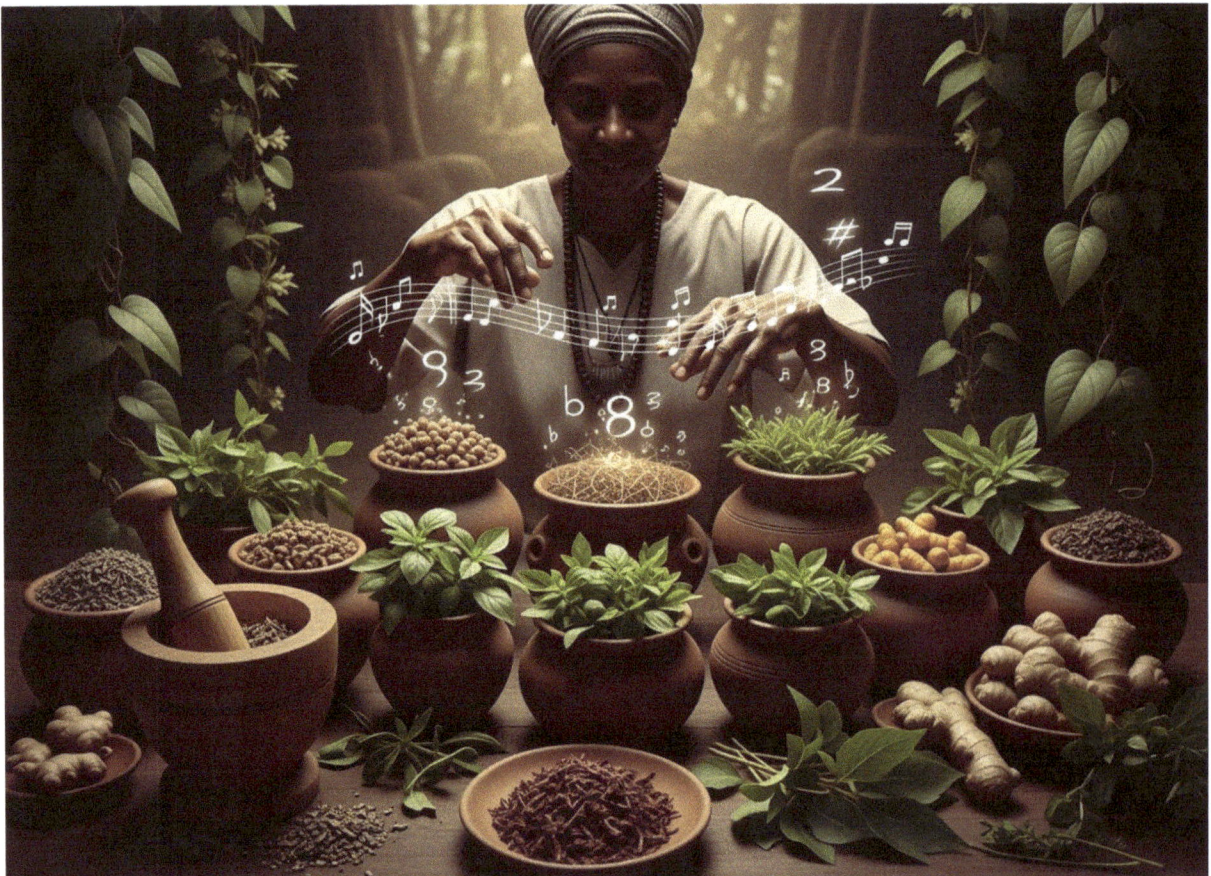

The Interconnected Web of Metabolism

Diabetes isn't just about blood sugar – it's a systemic metabolic disorder that affects every organ system. True healing requires rebalancing the entire metabolic symphony:

- **Liver function** (glucose production and storage)
- **Adrenal health** (stress hormone balance)
- **Thyroid optimization** (metabolic rate regulation)
- **Digestive restoration** (nutrient absorption)
- **Sleep quality** (hormone regulation)

Liver Support - The Metabolic Command Center

Your liver produces 75% of your body's glucose through a process called gluconeogenesis. In diabetes, the liver often produces excessive glucose, particularly at night, resulting in high morning blood sugar levels.

Milk Thistle (Silybum marianum)

- Protects liver cells from damage
- Improves glucose metabolism
- Reduces fatty liver (common in diabetics)
- Supports liver detoxification

Dosage: 200mg standardized extract (80% silymarin) twice daily

Adrenal Support - Stress and Blood Sugar

Chronic stress elevates cortisol, which in turn raises blood sugar levels and exacerbates insulin resistance. Supporting adrenal function is crucial for maintaining stable blood sugar levels.

Ashwagandha (Withania somnifera)

- Reduces cortisol levels by 30%
- Improves insulin sensitivity
- Reduces stress-related blood sugar spikes
- Supports overall energy and vitality

Dosage: 300mg twice daily (morning and evening)

Thyroid Support - The Metabolic Thermostat

Low thyroid function slows metabolism and worsens insulin resistance. Many diabetics have undiagnosed thyroid dysfunction.

Bladderwrack (Fucus vesiculosus)

- Provides natural iodine for thyroid function
- Boosts metabolic rate
- Supports weight management
- Provides essential trace minerals

Dosage: 500mg daily with breakfast

Digestive Support - The Foundation of Nutrition

Poor digestion can lead to nutrient deficiencies, which can worsen diabetes. Digestive enzymes help break down food properly and reduce post-meal blood sugar spikes.

Comprehensive Digestive Enzymes

- Amylase (breaks down carbohydrates)
- Protease (breaks down proteins)
- Lipase (breaks down fats)
- Additional enzymes for complete digestion

Dosage: 1-2 capsules with each meal

THE SYNERGISTIC EFFECT

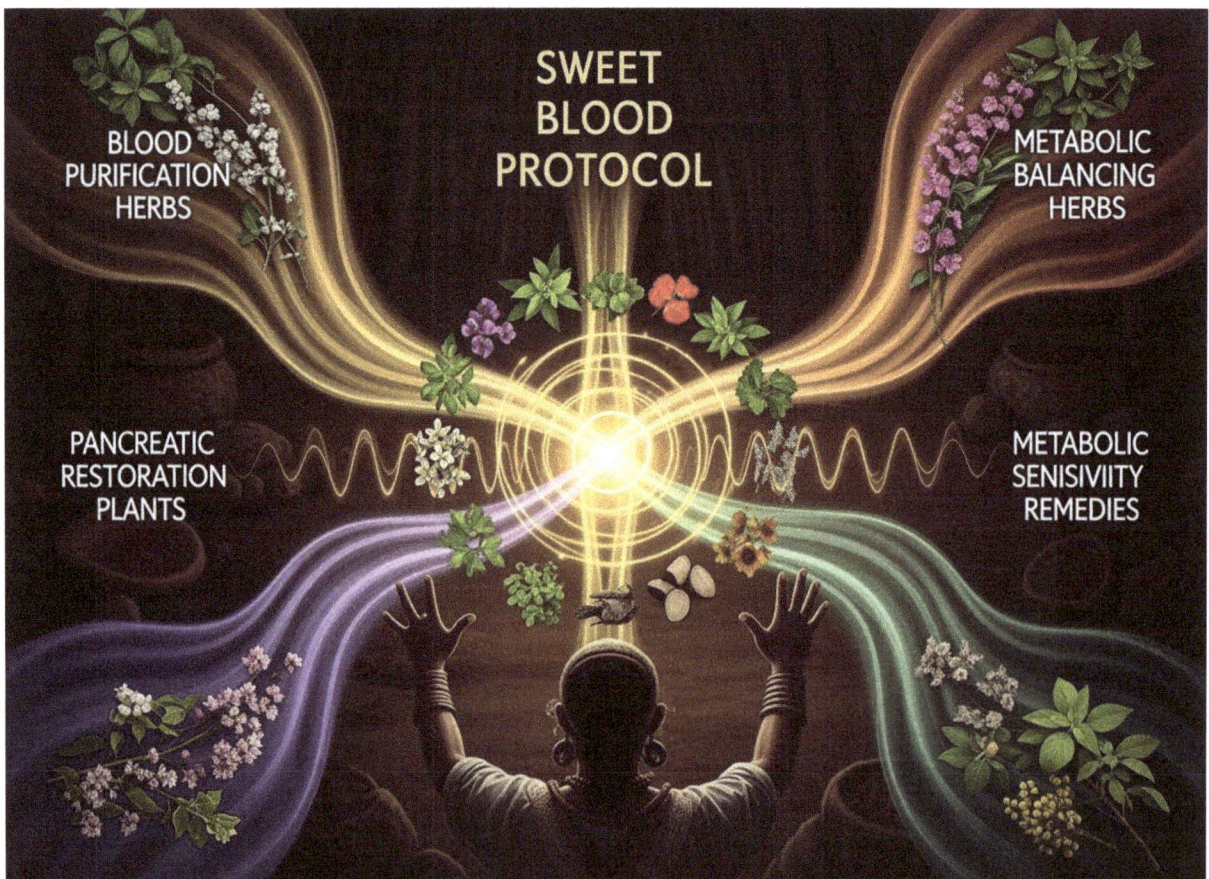

The magic of the Sweet Blood Protocol isn't in any single herb or supplement – it's in the synergistic interaction of all four pillars working together:

Pillar 1 (Blood Purification) creates the clean internal environment needed for healing. **Pillar 2 (Pancreatic Restoration)** rebuilds the organ that produces insulin. **Pillar 3 (Insulin Sensitivity Reset)** ensures cells can respond to insulin properly. **Pillar 4 (Metabolic Rebalancing)** optimizes all supporting systems

When all four pillars are implemented together, the result is a complete metabolic transformation – not just blood sugar control, but also the restoration of optimal health and vitality.

YOUR DAILY IMPLEMENTATION SCHEDULE

Morning (Upon Waking):

- Blood Purification Tea (8 oz)
- Bitter Melon Juice (2 oz) or extract (500mg)
- Chromium Picolinate (200mcg)
- Alpha-Lipoic Acid (300mg)
- Ashwagandha (300mg)

Pre-Breakfast (30 minutes before eating):

- Gymnema Sylvestre (400mg)
- Berberine (500mg)
- Digestive Enzymes (1-2 capsules)

Mid-Morning:

- Ceylon Cinnamon (500mg) or 1/2 tsp powder in tea

Pre-Lunch (30 minutes before eating):

- Chromium Picolinate (200mcg)
- Berberine (500mg)
- Digestive Enzymes (1-2 capsules)

Afternoon:

- Fenugreek Extract (300mg)
- Vanadyl Sulfate (10mg)

Pre-Dinner (30 minutes before eating):

- Chromium Picolinate (200mcg)
- Berberine (500mg)

- Digestive Enzymes (1-2 capsules)

Evening (Before Bed):

- Blood Purification Tea (8 oz)
- Alpha-Lipoic Acid (300mg)
- Milk Thistle (200mg)
- Ashwagandha (300mg)
- Vanadyl Sulfate (10mg)

Weekly:

- Bladderwrack (500mg daily)
- Comprehensive metabolic assessment
- Progress tracking and adjustments

MONITORING YOUR PROGRESS

Track these key indicators to monitor your transformation:

Daily Measurements:

- Morning fasting glucose
- Pre and post-meal readings
- Energy levels (1-10 scale)
- Sleep quality (1-10 scale)

Weekly Assessments:

- Weight and body measurements
- Overall well-being score
- Medication needs (with doctor supervision)
- Symptom improvements

Monthly Evaluations:

- A1C testing (every 3 months)
- Comprehensive metabolic panel
- Inflammation markers (CRP, ESR)
- Liver and kidney function

WHAT TO EXPECT

Week 1-2: Foundation Setting

- Initial blood sugar improvements

- Reduced sugar cravings
- Better sleep quality
- Increased energy·

Week 3-4: Momentum Building

- Consistent blood sugar improvements
- Possible medication adjustments needed
- Noticeable energy increases
- Mental clarity improvements

Week 6-8: Significant Progress

- Major blood sugar stabilization
- Potential medication reductions
- Weight loss begins
- Overall vitality returning

Week 10-12: Transformation Visible

- Near-normal blood sugar ranges
- Significant medication reductions
- Energy levels fully restored
- Confidence in health returning

Week 14-16: Diabetes Reversal

- A1C testing shows dramatic improvement
- Many people are completely off medications
- Full energy and vitality restored
- Diabetes reversal achieved

YOUR PERSONALIZED PROTOCOL

While these four pillars work for over 80% of people, individual customization may be needed based on your specific situation.

[Schedule Your FREE 15-Minute Consultation](#)

During this call, we'll:

- Assess your current health status
- Customize the protocol for your needs
- Address any concerns or questions
- Ensure you have everything needed for success

THE COMMITMENT TO HEALING

The Four Pillars of Diabetes Reversal represent more than just a treatment protocol – they represent a commitment to reclaiming your health and your life.

Each pillar requires dedication, consistency, and faith in your body's ability to heal. But when you commit fully to all four pillars, diabetes becomes not just manageable, but reversible.

In the next chapter, we'll dive into your Morning Ritual – the daily practice that sets the foundation for metabolic healing and diabetes reversal.

CHAPTER 7
YOUR MORNING RITUAL FOR METABOLIC RESET

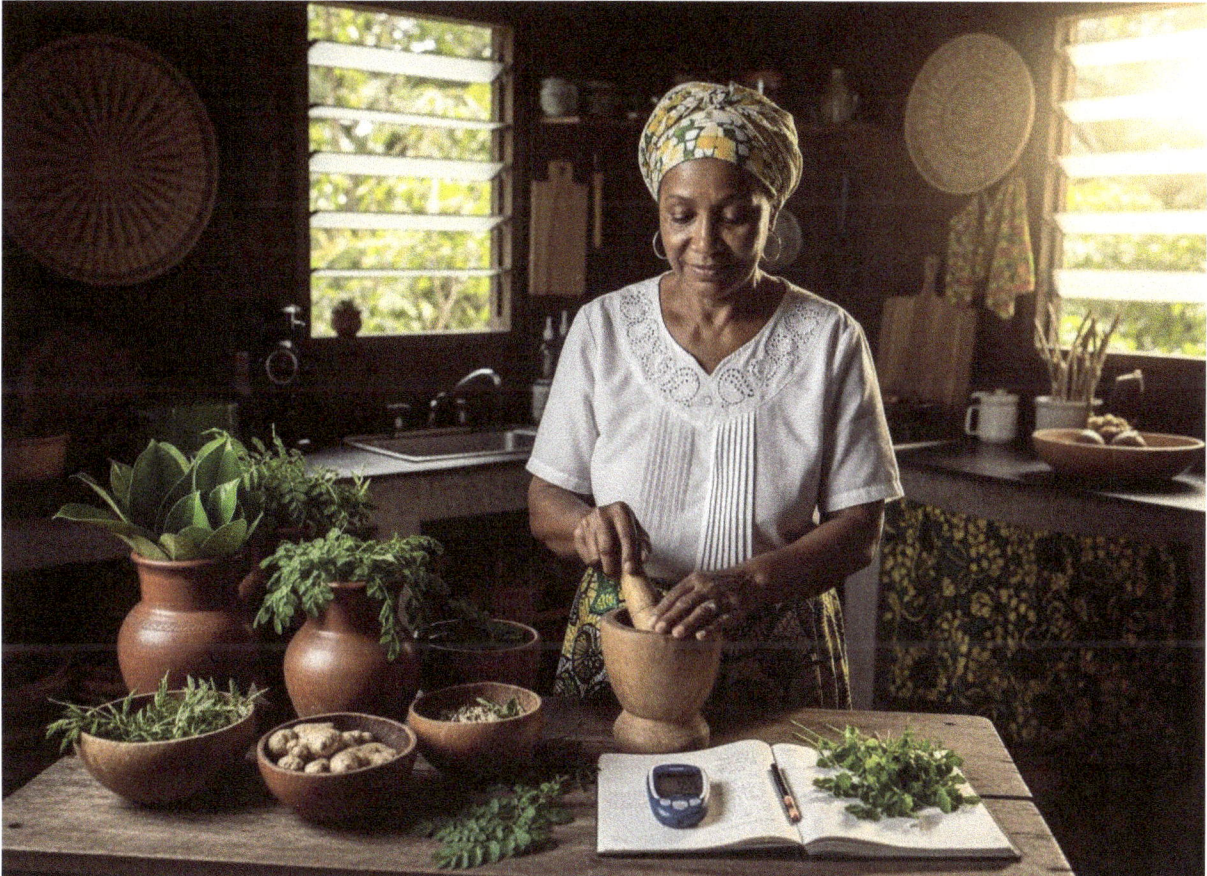

"How you start your morning determines how your metabolism functions all day. Master your morning ritual, and you master your blood sugar."

The first hour after waking is the most critical time for blood sugar control. During sleep, your liver produces glucose to fuel your brain and vital organs. How you break this overnight fast determines whether your blood sugar remains stable or spikes out of control.

The Morning Ritual isn't just about taking herbs – it's about creating a metabolic reset that optimizes your body's natural glucose regulation for the entire day.

THE SCIENCE OF MORNING METABOLISM

The Dawn Phenomenon occurs between 4-8 AM, when your body naturally releases hormones (cortisol, growth hormone, adrenaline) that raise blood sugar levels to prepare you for the day. In healthy individuals, the pancreas releases insulin to balance this rise. In diabetics, this system is disrupted, leading to high blood sugar levels in the morning.

The Somogyi Effect. Some diabetics experience overnight low blood sugar, triggering the release of counter-regulatory hormones that cause a rebound in high blood sugar in the morning. This creates a vicious cycle of unstable glucose levels.

The Metabolic Window The first 30-60 minutes after waking represent a critical metabolic window where the right interventions can reset your entire glucose regulation system for the day.

THE TRADITIONAL MORNING PROTOCOL

In the Blue Mountains of Jamaica, my ancestors began each day with a specific sequence of plant medicines designed to optimize metabolism and maintain stable blood sugar throughout the day.

This wasn't random folk medicine – it was a sophisticated understanding of circadian rhythms and metabolic function that modern science is only now beginning to validate.

YOUR COMPLETE MORNING RITUAL

STEP 1: HYDRATION AND ACTIVATION (Upon Waking)

Lemon Water Elixir: Before consuming anything else, drink 16 oz of warm water with:

- Juice of 1/2 fresh lemon
- 1/4 teaspoon Celtic sea salt
- 1 tablespoon apple cider vinegar

Why This Works:

- Rehydrates your body after 8 hours without water
- Lemon stimulates digestive enzymes and liver function
- Sea salt provides essential electrolytes
- Apple cider vinegar improves insulin sensitivity by 34%

STEP 2: BLOOD PURIFICATION TEA (15 minutes after lemon water)

The Master Morning Blend:

- Sarsaparilla Root: 1 teaspoon
- Burdock Root: 1 teaspoon
- Dandelion Root: 1/2 teaspoon
- Red Clover Blossoms: 1/2 teaspoon

Preparation:

1. Combine herbs in a tea strainer or French press
2. Pour 12 oz boiling water over herbs
3. Steep for 10 minutes
4. Strain and drink warm

Expected Effects:

- Deep cellular cleansing begins
- Liver detoxification pathways are activated
- Inflammatory markers begin to reduce
- Blood circulation improves

STEP 3: THE METABOLIC ACTIVATORS (With your tea)

Bitter Melon Extract - 500mg

- Provides plant insulin (polypeptide-p)
- Begins glucose regulation immediately
- Reduces morning blood sugar spikes
- Activates cellular glucose uptake

Chromium Picolinate - 200mcg

- Enhances insulin receptor sensitivity
- Improves glucose metabolism
- Reduces sugar cravings throughout the day
- Supports healthy weight management

Alpha-Lipoic Acid - 300mg

- Powerful antioxidant protection for pancreatic cells
- Improves glucose uptake by muscle cells
- Reduces oxidative stress from high blood sugar
- Supports nerve health and prevents neuropathy

Ashwagandha - 300mg

- Reduces morning cortisol levels by 30%
- Prevents stress-induced blood sugar spikes
- Supports adrenal function and energy production
- Improves overall stress resilience

STEP 4: THE PANCREATIC ACTIVATOR (30 minutes after tea)

Fresh Bitter Melon Juice - 2 oz If you can obtain fresh bitter melon (available at Asian markets), this is the most potent form of plant insulin available.

Preparation:

1. Wash 1 medium bitter melon
2. Cut lengthwise and remove seeds
3. Juice using a high-speed juicer
4. Drink immediately (can mix with a small amount of water)

Alternative: If fresh bitter melon isn't available, use standardized bitter melon extract (500mg) with 8 oz of water.

STEP 5: MOVEMENT AND ACTIVATION (45 minutes after waking)

Gentle Morning Movement. Before eating your first meal, engage in 10-15 minutes of gentle movement to activate glucose uptake by muscle cells:

- Light stretching or yoga
- Walking around your home or yard
- Simple calisthenics (arm circles, leg swings)
- Deep breathing exercises

Why Movement Matters:

- Increases insulin sensitivity by 40% for up to 24 hours
- Activates glucose transporters in muscle cells
- Reduces morning blood sugar naturally
- Improves circulation and energy levels

THE MORNING MEAL PROTOCOL

TIMING: Eat your first meal 60-90 minutes after waking, allowing the morning herbs to work first.

PRE-MEAL SUPPLEMENTS (30 minutes before eating):

Gymnema Sylvestre - 400mg

- Blocks sugar absorption in the intestines
- Reduces post-meal blood sugar spikes by 50%
- Eliminates sugar cravings
- Supports pancreatic beta cell regeneration

Berberine - 500mg

- Functions like natural metformin
- Reduces glucose production by the liver
- Improves insulin sensitivity
- Activates cellular energy pathways

Digestive Enzymes - 1-2 capsules

- Amylase for carbohydrate breakdown
- Protease for protein digestion
- Lipase for fat metabolism
- Reduces post-meal glucose spikes

OPTIMAL MORNING MEAL COMPOSITION

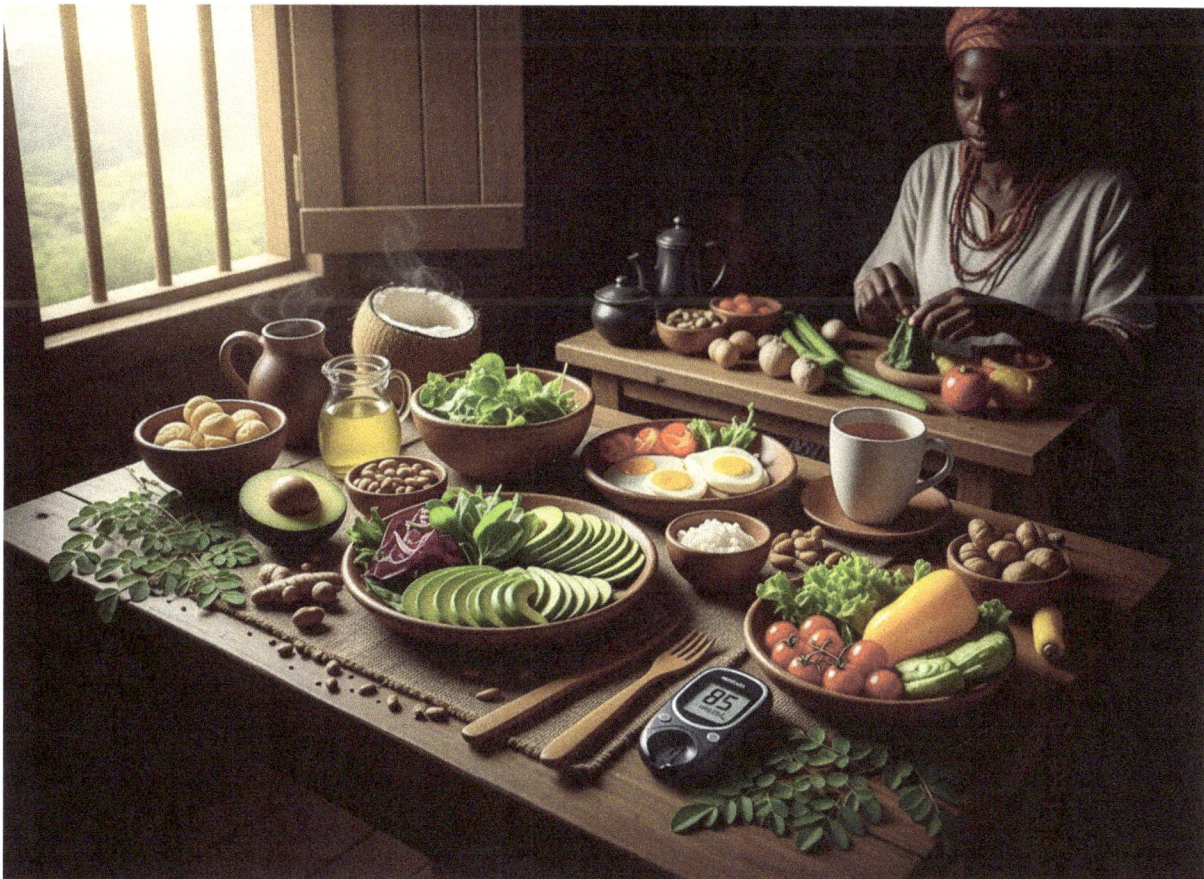

The 40-30-30 Formula:

- 40% healthy fats (avocado, nuts, seeds, olive oil)
- 30% quality protein (eggs, fish, organic poultry)
- 30% low-glycemic vegetables (leafy greens, cruciferous vegetables)

Sample Morning Meals:

Option 1: The Caribbean Scramble

- 2-3 eggs scrambled in coconut oil
- 1/2 avocado sliced
- Sautéed spinach and bell peppers
- 1 tablespoon ground flaxseed
- Sprinkle of Ceylon cinnamon

Option 2: The Green Power Bowl

- Large handful of mixed greens
- 1/4 cup raw almonds or walnuts
- 2 tablespoons hemp seeds
- 1/2 cucumber, diced
- 2 tablespoons olive oil and lemon dressing
- Optional: 3 oz wild-caught salmon

Option 3: The Metabolic Smoothie

- 1 cup unsweetened almond milk
- 1/2 avocado
- 1 cup spinach
- 1 tablespoon almond butter
- 1 tablespoon chia seeds
- 1/2 teaspoon Ceylon cinnamon
- Ice as needed

FOODS TO AVOID IN THE MORNING

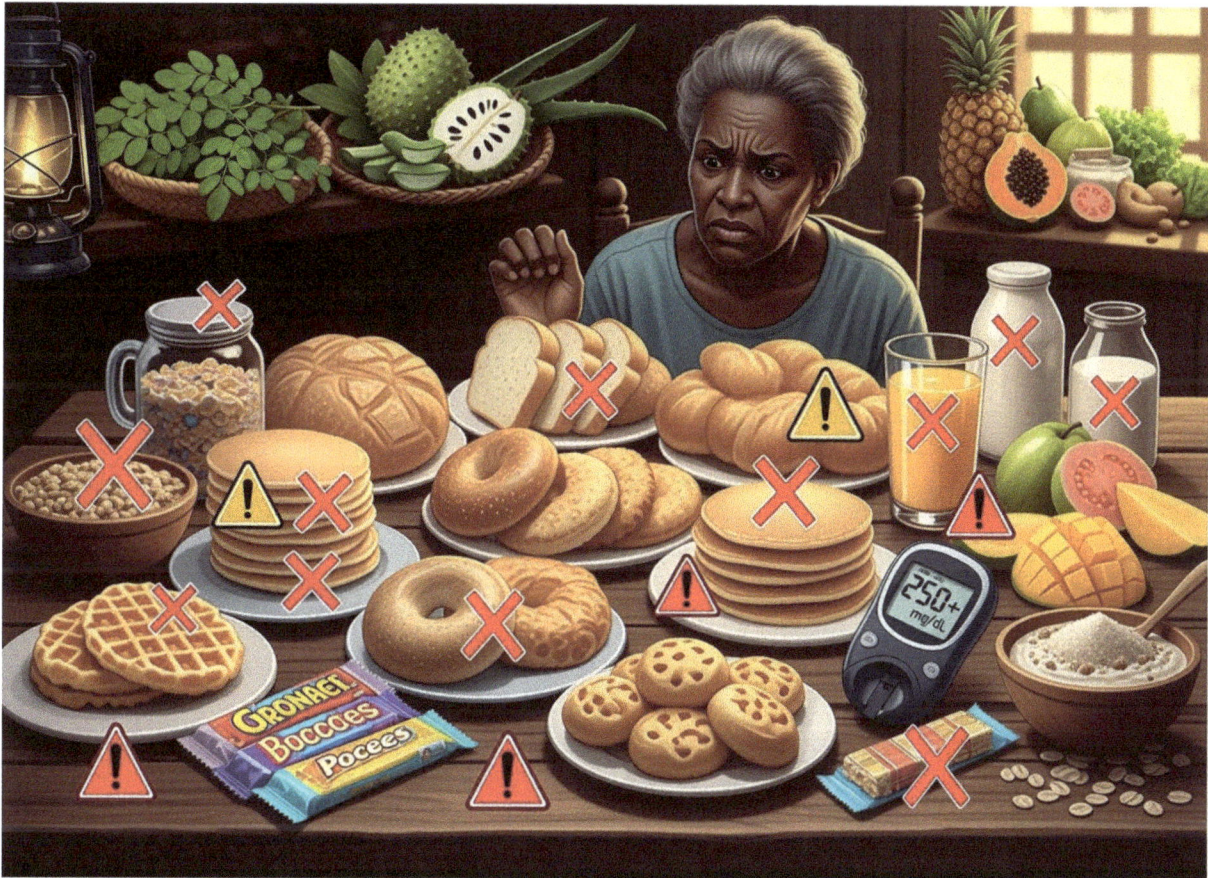

Never Start Your Day With:

- Cereals (even "healthy" ones)
- Bread, bagels, or pastries
- Fruit juices or smoothies with fruit
- Oatmeal or other grains
- Coffee with sugar or artificial sweeteners
- Processed breakfast foods

Why These Foods Sabotage Your Day:

- Causes immediate blood sugar spikes
- Trigger insulin resistance
- Create sugar cravings that last all day
- Disrupt metabolic balance
- Counteract the morning protocol benefits

THE COFFEE QUESTION

Can You Drink Coffee? Yes, but with important modifications:

Timing: Only after completing the morning ritual (at least 60 minutes after waking)

Preparation:

- Organic, mold-free coffee only
- Add 1 tablespoon MCT oil or coconut oil
- Add 1 tablespoon grass-fed butter (if tolerated)
- 1/4 teaspoon Ceylon cinnamon
- No sugar, artificial sweeteners, or regular milk

Why This Works:

- Healthy fats slow caffeine absorption
- MCT oil provides stable energy
- Cinnamon improves insulin sensitivity
- Avoids blood sugar spikes from additives

TRACKING YOUR MORNING SUCCESS

Daily Measurements: Record these metrics each morning:

Before Morning Ritual:

- Fasting blood glucose
- Energy level (1-10 scale)
- Mood assessment (1-10 scale)
- Sleep quality from the previous night (1-10 scale)

2 Hours After Morning Meal:

- Post-meal blood glucose
- Energy level (1-10 scale)
- Hunger/satiety level
- Any cravings or symptoms

Target Goals:

- Fasting glucose: 80-100 mg/dL
- Post-meal glucose: Under 140 mg/dL
- Energy level: 7-10 consistently
- No sugar cravings or energy crashes

TROUBLESHOOTING COMMON ISSUES

Problem: Morning blood sugar levels remain high after one week. Solution:

- Increase the bitter melon dose to 750mg
- Add 10mg vanadyl sulfate to morning supplements
- Extend fasting window to 14-16 hours
- Check for hidden stress or sleep issues

Problem: Feeling nauseous from morning herbs. Solution:

- Take supplements with a small amount of food
- Reduce alpha-lipoic acid to 200mg initially
- Dilute bitter melon juice with more water
- Start with half doses and gradually increase

Problem: No energy improvement. Solution:

- Check thyroid function (TSH, T3, T4)
- Add B-complex vitamins to morning routine
- Ensure adequate sleep (7-9 hours nightly)
- Consider adrenal fatigue assessment

Problem: Still craving sugar in the morning. Solution:

- Increase gymnema sylvestre to 600mg
- Add chromium picolinate dose (total 400mcg)
- Ensure adequate protein in the morning meal
- Check for emotional eating triggers

THE 21-DAY MORNING RITUAL CHALLENGE

Week 1: Foundation Building

- Focus on consistency with basic ritual
- Track blood sugar and energy levels
- Adjust timing and doses as needed
- Build the habit of morning movement

Week 2: Optimization

- Fine-tune supplement timing and doses
- Experiment with different morning meals
- Add coffee protocol if desired
- Notice improvements in energy and cravings

Week 3: Mastery

- Morning ritual becomes automatic
- Blood sugar stability improves significantly
- Energy levels are consistently high
- Reduced dependence on medications (with doctor supervision)

REAL SUCCESS STORIES

Maria's Morning Transformation: "I used to wake up with blood sugars over 200 every morning, no matter what I did. After just one week of the morning ritual, my fasting glucose dropped to 150. By week three, I was consistently waking up between 90-110. The bitter melon juice was hard to get used to, but the results speak for themselves."

James's Energy Revolution: "For years, I needed three cups of coffee just to function in the morning. The morning ritual gave me natural energy I hadn't felt in decades. My blood sugars stabilized, and I actually look forward to getting up now instead of dreading another day of managing diabetes."

YOUR PERSONALIZED MORNING PROTOCOL

While this morning ritual works for most people, individual customization may be needed based on:

- Current medications and timing
- Work schedule and lifestyle
- Food preferences and tolerances
- Severity of diabetes and other health conditions

[Schedule Your FREE 15-Minute Consultation](#)

During this call, we'll customize your morning ritual to fit your specific needs and ensure maximum effectiveness for your situation.

THE RIPPLE EFFECT

The Morning Ritual creates a positive ripple effect that influences your entire day:

Immediate Effects (0-2 hours):

- Stable blood sugar levels
- Sustained energy without crashes
- Reduced sugar cravings
- Mental clarity and focus

Daily Effects (2-12 hours):

- Better food choices throughout the day
- Improved insulin sensitivity
- Stable mood and energy
- Better stress resilience

Long-term Effects (weeks to months):

- Significant A1C improvements
- Reduced medication needs
- Weight loss and better body composition
- Overall health transformation

THE SACRED START

Your morning ritual is more than just a health protocol – it's a sacred start to each day that honors your commitment to healing and transformation.

Each morning, as you prepare your blood purification tea and take your metabolic activators, you're connecting with 300 years of healing wisdom and joining thousands of others who have found freedom from diabetes.

This ritual represents hope, healing, and the unshakeable belief that your body can restore itself when given the right tools.

In the next chapter, we'll explore your Midday Activation protocol – the strategies that maintain stable blood sugar and sustained energy throughout your most active hours.

CHAPTER 8
MIDDAY ACTIVATION AND
BLOOD SUGAR CONTROL

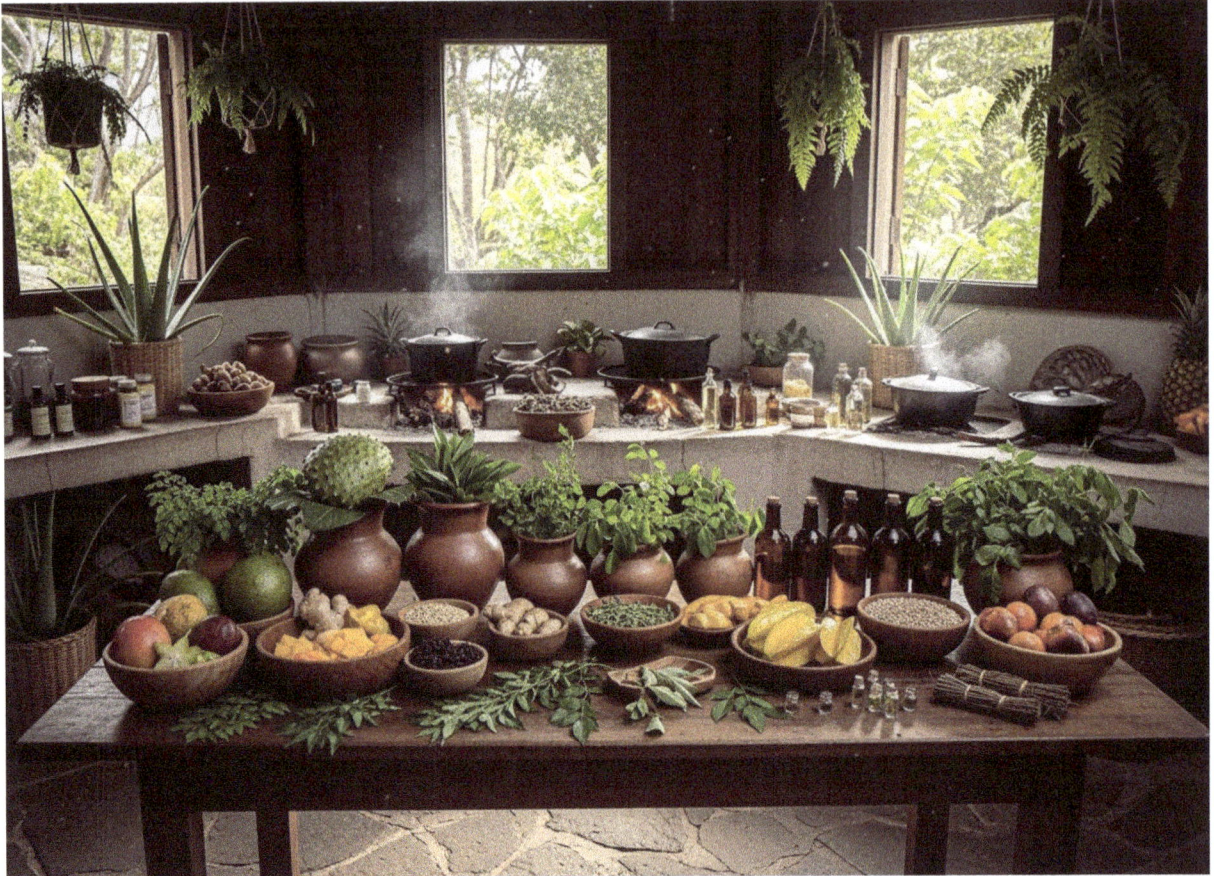

"The midday hours are when most diabetics lose control of their blood sugar. Master your midday protocol, and you master your diabetes."

Between 11 AM and 4 PM, your body faces its greatest metabolic challenges. This is when most people eat their largest meal, experience the highest stress levels, and make the food choices that either support healing or sabotage progress.

The Midday Activation Protocol isn't just about managing lunch – it's about maintaining the metabolic momentum created by your morning ritual and setting yourself up for stable blood sugar throughout the afternoon and evening.

THE MIDDAY METABOLIC CHALLENGE

The Post-Lunch Crisis. For most diabetics, the 2-4 PM period represents a metabolic disaster. Blood sugars spike from lunch, energy crashes from insulin surges, and sugar cravings intensify as glucose levels fluctuate wildly.

This isn't inevitable – it's the result of poor meal timing, incorrect food combinations, and lack of metabolic support during your body's most active period.

Stress and Blood Sugar. Midday is typically when work stress, family demands, and daily pressures peak. Stress hormones, such as cortisol, directly raise blood sugar levels, often causing spikes that are unrelated to food intake.

The Digestive Fire. Traditional medicine recognizes that digestive power is strongest between 10 AM and 2 PM. This is when your body can most effectively process nutrients and maintain stable blood sugar – if you know how to work with these natural rhythms.

THE TRADITIONAL MIDDAY WISDOM

My Maroon ancestors understood that midday required different plant medicines than those used in the morning or evening. They developed specific protocols for maintaining energy and blood sugar stability during the most active part of the day.

These weren't just random herbs – they were carefully selected plants that support sustained energy, mental clarity, and metabolic balance during peak activity hours.

YOUR COMPLETE MIDDAY ACTIVATION PROTOCOL

PRE-LUNCH PREPARATION (30 minutes before eating)

The Glucose Control Trio:

Gymnema Sylvestre - 400mg

- Blocks up to 50% of sugar absorption in the intestines
- Reduces post-meal glucose spikes dramatically
- Eliminates sugar cravings for 2-4 hours
- Supports pancreatic beta cell regeneration

White Mulberry Leaf Extract - 300mg

- Contains DNJ (1-deoxynojirimycin) that blocks carbohydrate absorption
- Reduces post-meal blood sugar by 40%
- Slows gastric emptying for sustained satiety
- Provides antioxidant protection

Berberine - 500mg

- Activates the AMPK pathway for improved glucose metabolism
- Reduces glucose production by the liver during meals
- Improves insulin sensitivity by 45%
- Functions like natural metformin without side effects

The Digestive Support Complex:

Comprehensive Digestive Enzymes - 2 capsules

- Amylase: Breaks down complex carbohydrates slowly
- Protease: Ensures complete protein digestion
- Lipase: Optimizes fat metabolism and absorption
- Additional enzymes: Support complete nutrient breakdown

Apple Cider Vinegar - 1 tablespoon in 8 oz water

- Improves insulin sensitivity by 34%
- Slows gastric emptying and carbohydrate absorption
- Reduces post-meal glucose spikes by 25%
- Supports healthy pH balance for optimal digestion

THE OPTIMAL MIDDAY MEAL STRUCTURE

The 50-25-25 Formula for Lunch:

- 50% non-starchy vegetables (variety of colors and textures)
- 25% quality protein (palm-sized portion)
- 25% healthy fats (avocado, nuts, olive oil, seeds)

Carbohydrate Guidelines:

- Limit total carbohydrates to 15-20 grams
- Choose only low-glycemic options (leafy greens, cruciferous vegetables)
- Avoid all grains, starches, and sugars
- Include fiber-rich vegetables to slow absorption

POWER LUNCH OPTIONS

Option 1: The Mediterranean Bowl

- 2 cups mixed greens (arugula, spinach, romaine)
- 4 oz grilled wild salmon
- 1/2 avocado, sliced
- 1/4 cup raw walnuts
- 2 tablespoons extra virgin olive oil
- 1 tablespoon lemon juice
- Fresh herbs (basil, oregano)

Estimated Impact: Blood sugar rise <20 mg/dL, sustained energy for 4+ hours

Option 2: The Asian-Inspired Stir-Fry

- 2 cups mixed vegetables (broccoli, bell peppers, snap peas)
- 4 oz organic chicken thigh, cubed
- 1 tablespoon of coconut oil for cooking
- 2 tablespoons raw almonds
- Ginger, garlic, and herbs for flavor
- 1 tablespoon coconut aminos (soy sauce alternative)

Estimated Impact: Blood sugar rise <15 mg/dL, mental clarity maintained

Option 3: The Protein Power Salad

- 3 cups baby spinach and kale mix
- 2 hard-boiled eggs, sliced
- 2 oz grass-fed beef or turkey, sliced
- 1/4 cup pumpkin seeds
- 1/2 cucumber, diced
- 2 tablespoons avocado oil dressing

- Fresh herbs and spices

Estimated Impact: Blood sugar rise <10 mg/dL, appetite satisfied for hours

POST-MEAL ACTIVATION PROTOCOL

Immediately After Eating:

Ceylon Cinnamon - 500mg or 1/2 teaspoon powder

- Improves insulin sensitivity by 40%
- Reduces post-meal glucose spikes
- Mimics insulin action in muscle cells
- Provides antioxidant protection

Chromium Picolinate - 200mcg

- Enhances glucose uptake by cells
- Improves insulin receptor function
- Reduces afternoon sugar cravings
- Supports healthy weight management

15-20 Minutes After Eating:

Gentle Movement Protocol: Never underestimate the power of post-meal movement for blood sugar control:

- 10-15 minute walk (even around the office)
- Light stretching or desk exercises
- Stair climbing if available
- Simple bodyweight movements

Why This Works:

- Increases glucose uptake by muscle cells by 30%
- Reduces post-meal blood sugar spikes significantly
- Improves insulin sensitivity for hours
- Prevents afternoon energy crashes

THE AFTERNOON ENERGY MAINTENANCE

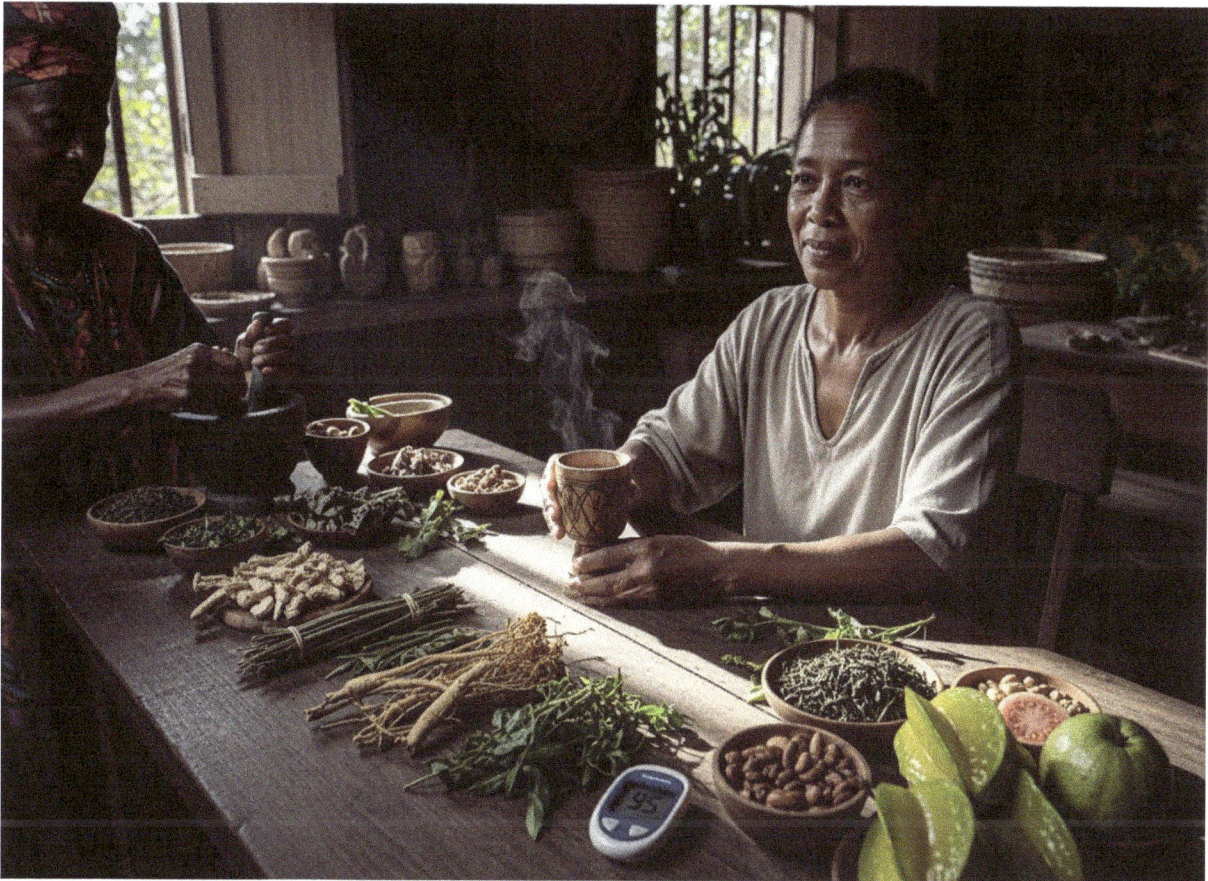

2 PM Support Protocol:

Green Tea Extract - 200mg EGCG

- Provides sustained energy without jitters
- Improves insulin sensitivity
- Supports fat metabolism
- Provides powerful antioxidant protection

L-Theanine - 100mg

- Promotes calm, focused energy
- Reduces stress-induced blood sugar spikes
- Improves mental clarity without stimulation
- Balances cortisol levels naturally

Alpha-Lipoic Acid - 300mg

- Continuous glucose uptake support
- Provides ongoing antioxidant protection

- Supports nerve health and circulation
- Maintains insulin sensitivity

STRESS MANAGEMENT FOR BLOOD SUGAR CONTROL

The Stress-Glucose Connection Stress hormones (cortisol, adrenaline, norepinephrine) can raise blood sugar by 50-100 mg/dL within minutes, regardless of food intake. Managing midday stress is crucial for diabetes reversal.

The 5-Minute Reset Protocol:

Deep Breathing Exercise:

1. Inhale for 4 counts through the nose
2. Hold breath for 4 counts
3. Exhale for 6 counts through the mouth
4. Repeat 10 times

Progressive Muscle Relaxation:

1. Tense shoulders for 5 seconds, then release
2. Clench fists for 5 seconds, then release
3. Tighten facial muscles for 5 seconds, then release
4. Feel the wave of relaxation throughout the body

Mindful Moment:

1. Focus on 3 things you can see
2. Notice 2 things you can hear
3. Identify 1 thing you can smell
4. Take 3 deep, grateful breaths

HYDRATION AND ELECTROLYTE BALANCE

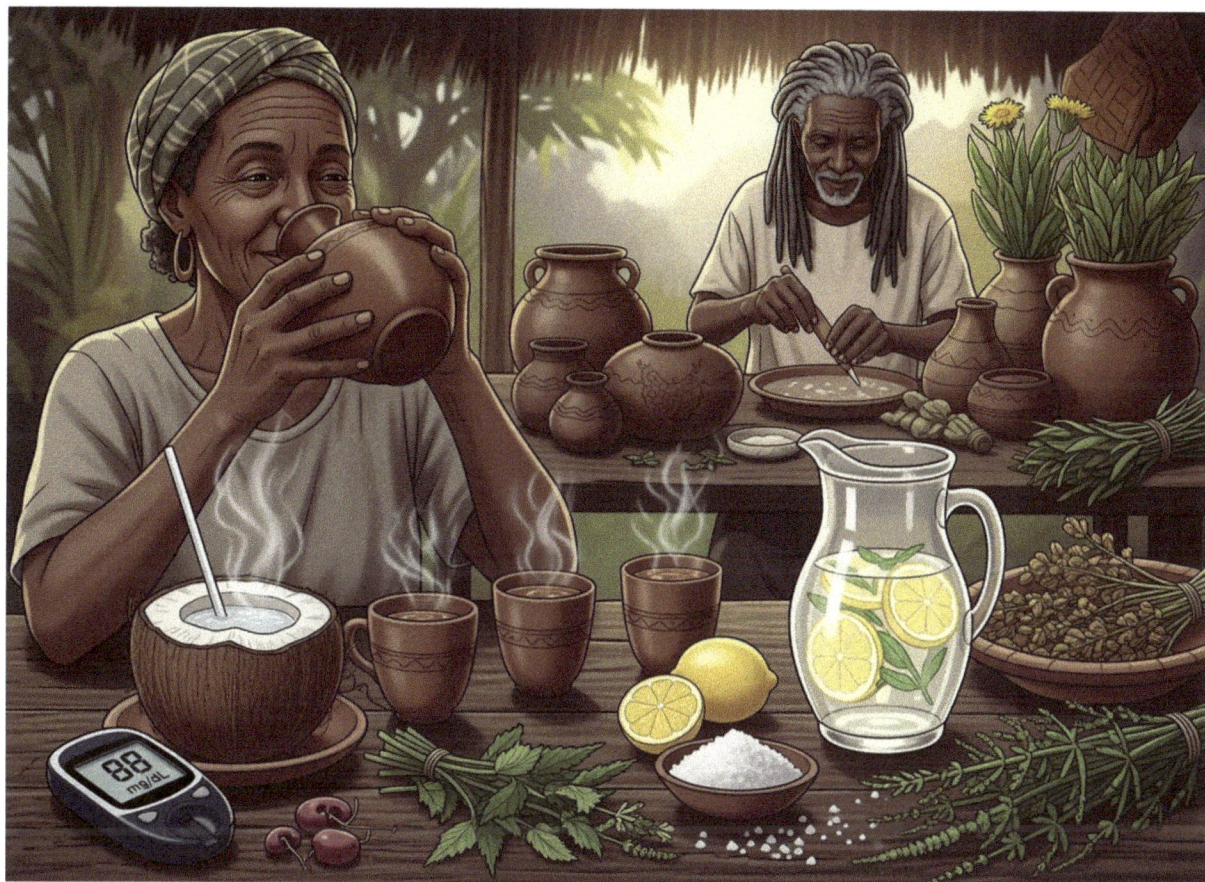

The Midday Hydration Protocol:

Between Meals (every 2 hours):

- 8-12 oz filtered water
- Pinch of Himalayan sea salt
- Squeeze of fresh lemon
- Optional: 1/4 teaspoon apple cider vinegar

Why This Matters:

- Dehydration raises blood sugar by concentrating glucose
- Proper electrolyte balance supports insulin function
- Lemon provides vitamin C and supports liver function
- ACV continues to improve insulin sensitivity

AVOIDING THE AFTERNOON CRASH

Common Midday Mistakes:

- Eating too many carbohydrates at lunch
- Skipping the pre-meal supplement protocol
- Not moving after eating
- Drinking sugary beverages or diet sodas
- Eating processed "healthy" snacks

The Energy Sustaining Strategy:

- Follow the 50-25-25 meal formula strictly
- Take all pre-meal supplements as directed
- Include 15 minutes of post-meal movement
- Stay properly hydrated with electrolytes
- Manage stress proactively

EMERGENCY BLOOD SUGAR PROTOCOLS

If Blood Sugar Spikes Above 200 mg/dL:

Immediate Actions:

1. Drink 16 oz of water with 1 tablespoon of apple cider vinegar
2. Take an additional 400mg of gymnema sylvestre
3. Walk for 20-30 minutes if possible
4. Practice deep breathing exercises
5. Recheck blood sugar in 1 hour

If Blood Sugar Drops Below 70 mg/dL:

1. Consume 15g fast-acting carbs (4 oz orange juice)
2. Recheck in 15 minutes
3. If still low, repeat with another 15g of carbs
4. Once stable, eat a small protein/fat snack
5. Assess what caused the low (too much medication, not enough food, etc.)

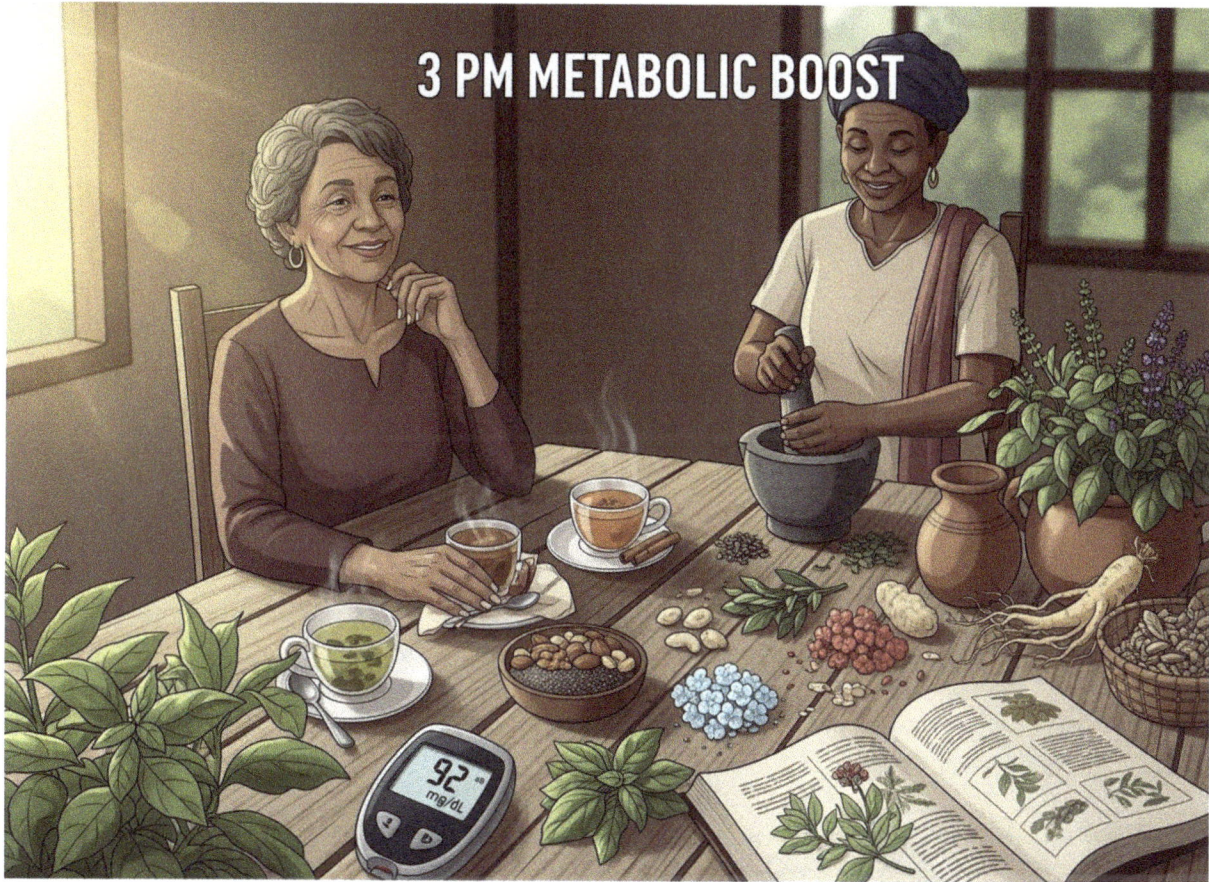

3 PM METABOLIC BOOST

The Traditional Caribbean Pick-Me-Up:

Herbal Energy Tea Blend:

- Green tea: 1 teaspoon
- Ginseng root: 1/2 teaspoon
- Ginger root: 1/4 teaspoon
- Ceylon cinnamon: 1/4 teaspoon
- Steep 10 minutes, strain, drink warm

Benefits:

- Natural energy without blood sugar spikes
- Improved mental clarity and focus
- Continued insulin sensitivity support
- Stress reduction and mood enhancement

SOCIAL EATING STRATEGIES

Business Lunches and Social Meals:

Restaurant Survival Guide:

- Review the menu online beforehand
- Take pre-meal supplements in the car/bathroom
- Order first to avoid peer pressure
- Ask for substitutions confidently
- Focus on protein and vegetables
- Request dressing/sauces on the side

Sample Restaurant Orders:

- Grilled salmon with steamed broccoli (no rice)
- Chicken Caesar salad (no croutons, dressing on side)
- Steak with side salad and avocado
- Vegetable omelet with a side of mixed greens

Social Pressure Management:

- "I'm following a specific health protocol."
- "My doctor has me on a special diet."
- "I feel so much better eating this way."
- "I'm not hungry for dessert, but thank you."

TRACKING MIDDAY SUCCESS

Key Metrics to Monitor:

Pre-Lunch:

- Blood glucose level
- Hunger level (1-10 scale)
- Energy level (1-10 scale)
- Stress level (1-10 scale)

2 Hours Post-Lunch:

- Blood glucose level
- Energy level (sustained vs. crashed)
- Mental clarity and focus
- Any cravings or symptoms

Target Goals:

- Post-meal glucose rise: <40 mg/dL
- Energy level: 7-10 consistently
- No afternoon crashes or cravings
- Mental clarity maintained

TROUBLESHOOTING MIDDAY CHALLENGES

Problem: Still getting afternoon energy crashes. Solutions:

- Reduce carbohydrates at lunch to <15g
- Increase healthy fats to 30% of the meal
- Add 200mg of additional chromium
- Ensure 20 minutes post-meal movement

Problem: Blood sugar levels spike despite taking supplements. Solutions:

- Take supplements 45 minutes before eating
- Increase gymnema sylvestre to 600mg
- Add 300mg white mulberry leaf extract
- Check for hidden carbs in foods

Problem: Intense sugar cravings at 3 PM. Solutions:

- Increase protein at lunch
- Add 100mg L-theanine for stress
- Drink herbal energy tea instead of snacking
- Practice 5-minute reset protocol

Problem: Difficulty with social eating situations. Solutions:

- Eat a small protein snack before social meals
- Take a double dose of pre-meal supplements
- Focus on socializing rather than food
- Plan your order strategy in advance

REAL SUCCESS STORIES

David's Midday Transformation: "I used to crash every afternoon around 2 PM. My blood sugar would spike to 250 after lunch, then I'd be exhausted and craving sugar all afternoon. The midday protocol changed everything. Now my post-meal readings stay under 140, and I have steady energy all day long."

Valh's Social Eating Victory: "Business lunches were sabotaging my progress. I learned to take my supplements beforehand and order strategically. Last week, I had three business meals, and my blood sugars never went above 130. My colleagues are asking what my secret is!"

THE MIDDAY MOMENTUM

The Midday Activation Protocol creates momentum that carries you through the rest of your day:

Immediate Benefits (1-4 hours):

- Stable blood sugar after meals
- Sustained energy without crashes
- Mental clarity and focus
- Reduced sugar cravings

Daily Benefits (affects evening and night):

- Better food choices at dinner
- Improved sleep quality
- Stable overnight blood sugars
- Morning readings in the normal range

Long-term Benefits (weeks to months):

- Consistent A1C improvements
- Reduced medication needs
- Better stress management
- Overall metabolic health

YOUR PERSONALIZED MIDDAY STRATEGY

Every person's midday challenges are different based on:

- Work schedule and environment
- Social eating requirements
- Stress levels and triggers
- Current medications and timing

[Schedule Your FREE 15-Minute Consultation](#)

During this call, we'll customize your midday protocol to address your specific challenges and ensure maximum blood sugar control during your most active hours.

THE POWER OF CONSISTENCY

The Midday Activation Protocol isn't about perfection – it's about consistency. Each day that you follow the protocol, you're:

- Reinforcing healthy metabolic patterns
- Building insulin sensitivity
- Creating sustainable habits
- Moving closer to diabetes reversal

Even when social situations or work demands disrupt your routine, the core principles remain the same: pre-meal supplements, smart food choices, post-meal movement, and stress management.

THE BRIDGE TO EVENING

Your midday protocol sets the stage for a successful evening. When you maintain stable blood sugar and sustained energy throughout the afternoon, you're more likely to:

- Make healthy dinner choices
- Have energy for evening activities
- Sleep better and wake refreshed
- Start the next day with optimal blood sugar

In the next chapter, we'll explore your Evening Restoration protocol – the practices that support overnight healing and ensure you wake up with stable blood sugar.

CHAPTER 9
EVENING RESTORATION AND CELLULAR REPAIR

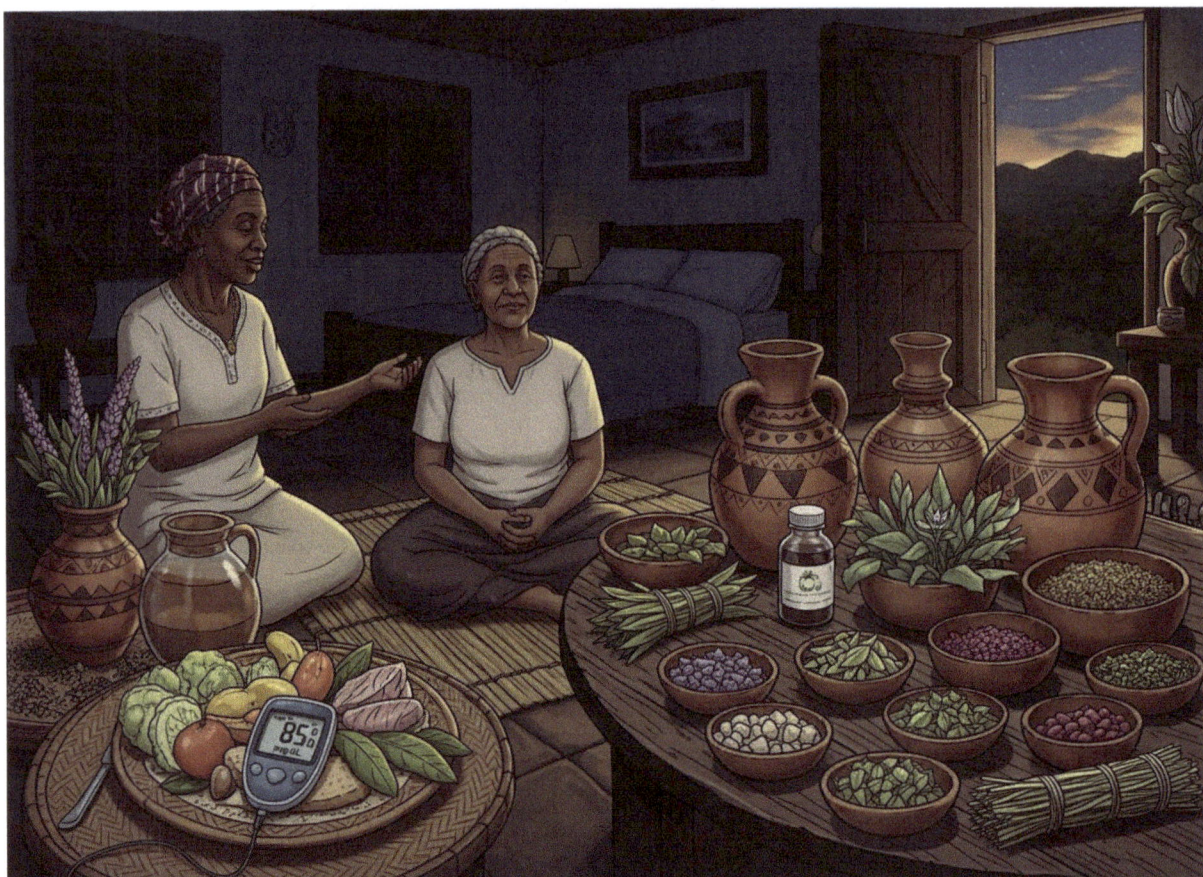

"The evening hours are when your body shifts from active metabolism to healing and repair. Master your evening protocol, and you wake up renewed and restored."

As the sun sets and your body prepares for rest, a remarkable transformation occurs. Your metabolism shifts from the active, energy-demanding processes of the day to the restorative, healing functions of night.

For diabetics, the evening hours represent both the greatest opportunity for healing and the highest risk for metabolic disruption. Get your evening protocol right, and you'll wake up with stable blood sugar and renewed energy. Get it wrong, and you'll start tomorrow already behind.

THE SCIENCE OF EVENING METABOLISM

The Circadian Rhythm Connection: Your body operates on a 24-hour circadian rhythm that affects every aspect of metabolism. As evening approaches, several critical changes occur:

- Insulin sensitivity naturally decreases by 20-30%
- Growth hormone production increases for tissue repair
- Cortisol levels should drop to allow restorative sleep
- The liver switches from glucose storage to glucose production
- Cellular repair and detoxification processes activate

The Evening Insulin Challenge: Between 6 PM and midnight, your body becomes naturally more insulin resistant. This evolutionary adaptation helped our ancestors store energy for the overnight fast, but in modern diabetics, it can cause dangerous blood sugar elevations.

The Overnight Glucose Production During sleep, your liver produces glucose to fuel your brain and vital organs. In healthy individuals, this process is tightly regulated. In diabetics, excessive glucose production can cause morning blood sugar spikes.

THE TRADITIONAL EVENING WISDOM

My Maroon ancestors understood that evening required different plant medicines than those used in the morning or midday. They developed specific protocols to support the body's natural transition from activity to rest, ensuring stable blood sugar levels throughout the night.

These evening rituals weren't just about blood sugar control – they were about supporting the deep cellular repair that happens during sleep, the process that ultimately reverses diabetes at the cellular level.

YOUR COMPLETE EVENING RESTORATION PROTOCOL

EARLY EVENING PREPARATION (5-6 PM)

The Metabolic Transition Support:

Milk Thistle Extract - 200mg

- Supports liver detoxification processes
- Prepares the liver for overnight glucose regulation
- Protects against oxidative stress
- Reduces fatty liver associated with diabetes

Magnesium Glycinate - 400mg

- Improves insulin sensitivity by 25%
- Supports muscle relaxation and stress reduction
- Essential for over 300 enzymatic processes
- Promotes deeper, more restorative sleep

Omega-3 Fatty Acids - 1000mg EPA/DHA

- Reduces inflammation throughout the body
- Improves insulin sensitivity
- Supports brain health and mood
- Essential for cellular membrane function

THE OPTIMAL EVENING MEAL PROTOCOL

TIMING: Eat your final meal 3-4 hours before bedtime to allow complete digestion before sleep.

PRE-DINNER SUPPLEMENTS (30 minutes before eating):

The Evening Glucose Control Trio:

Gymnema Sylvestre - 400mg

- Blocks sugar absorption for the evening meal
- Reduces post-dinner glucose spikes
- Eliminates evening sugar cravings
- Supports overnight blood sugar stability

Berberine - 500mg

- Reduces liver glucose production overnight
- Improves insulin sensitivity for the evening meal
- Activates cellular repair pathways
- Functions as a natural metformin

Digestive Enzymes - 2 capsules

- Ensures complete digestion before sleep
- Reduces overnight digestive stress
- Prevents blood sugar fluctuations from poor digestion
- Supports nutrient absorption for healing

EVENING MEAL COMPOSITION

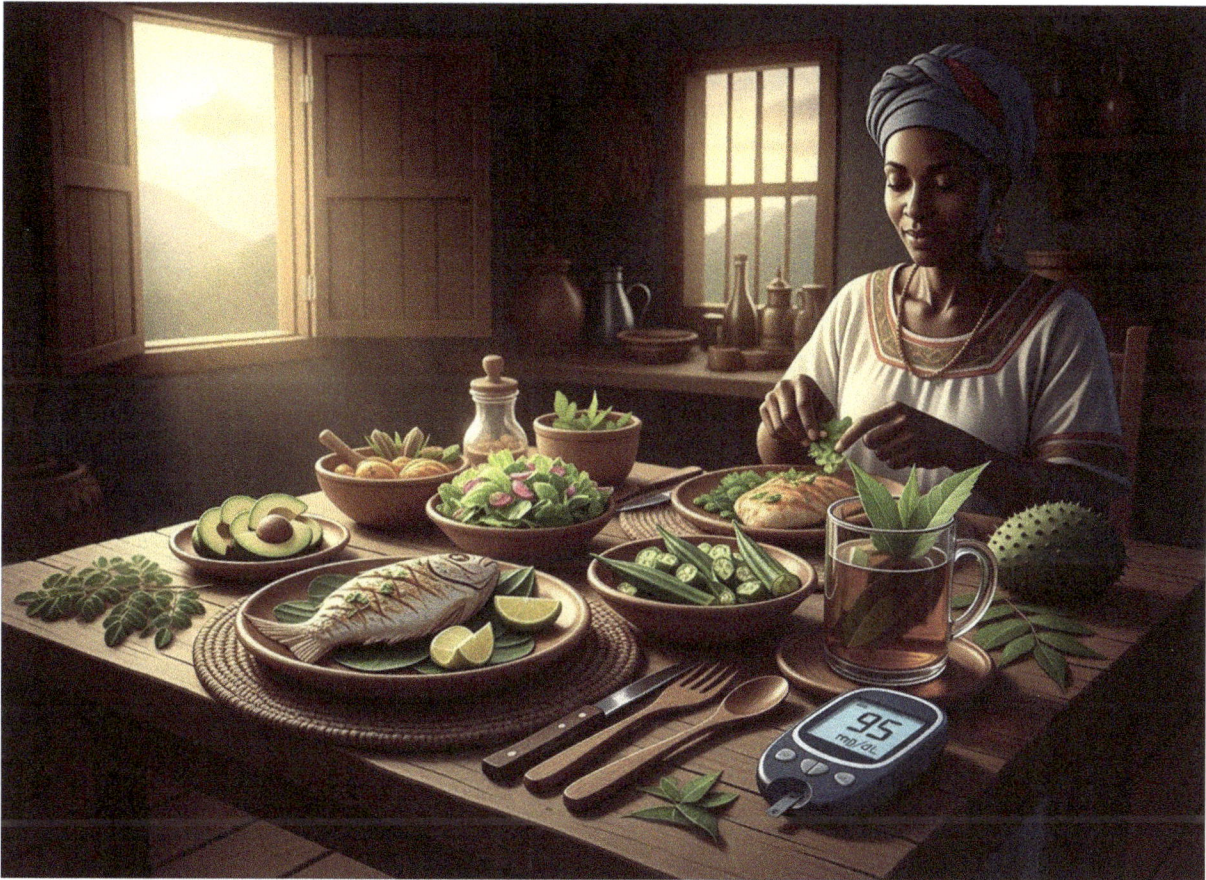

The 60-25-15 Evening Formula:

- 60% non-starchy vegetables (emphasizing leafy greens)
- 25% quality protein (slightly less than lunch)
- 15% healthy fats (lighter than midday meal)

Evening Meal Principles:

- Lighter than lunch but satisfying
- Emphasize easily digestible proteins
- Include magnesium-rich vegetables
- Avoid all stimulating foods and spices
- No carbohydrates except low-glycemic vegetables

RESTORATIVE DINNER OPTIONS

Option 1: The Mediterranean Evening Bowl

- 2 cups mixed greens (spinach, arugula, romaine)
- 3 oz wild-caught cod or halibut

- 1/4 avocado, sliced
- 2 tablespoons pumpkin seeds
- Steamed asparagus and zucchini
- 1 tablespoon olive oil and lemon dressing

Estimated Impact: Minimal blood sugar rise, promotes restful sleep

Option 2: The Comfort Healing Soup

- Bone broth base with organic vegetables
- 3 oz shredded organic chicken
- Sautéed kale, spinach, and celery
- 1 tablespoon coconut oil
- Fresh herbs (parsley, thyme, oregano)
- Sea salt and pepper to taste

Estimated Impact: Deeply nourishing, supports overnight repair

Option 3: The Garden Fresh Plate

- Large mixed green salad with herbs
- 2 hard-boiled eggs, sliced
- Steamed broccoli and Brussels sprouts
- 2 tablespoons raw almonds
- Avocado oil and herb dressing
- Fresh cucumber and radishes

Estimated Impact: Light, digestible, blood sugar stable

POST-DINNER ACTIVATION (Immediately after eating)

Ceylon Cinnamon - 500mg

- Improves insulin sensitivity for the evening meal
- Helps regulate overnight glucose production
- Provides antioxidant protection during sleep
- Supports healthy blood pressure

Vanadyl Sulfate - 10mg

- Mimics insulin action overnight
- Reduces morning blood sugar spikes
- Supports glucose uptake by muscle cells
- Helps maintain stable overnight levels

Gentle Evening Movement (15-20 minutes after dinner):

- Leisurely walk around the neighborhood
- Light stretching or gentle yoga
- Tai chi or qigong movements
- Simple household activities

Why Evening Movement Matters:

- Reduces post-dinner blood sugar spikes by 30%
- Improves overnight insulin sensitivity
- Supports healthy digestion before sleep
- Reduces stress and promotes relaxation

THE EVENING WIND-DOWN RITUAL (7-8 PM)

Blood Purification Evening Tea:

The Restorative Blend:

- Chamomile flowers: 1 teaspoon (calming, sleep-promoting)
- Dandelion root: 1/2 teaspoon (liver support, detoxification)
- Red clover blossoms: 1/2 teaspoon (blood cleansing)
- Passionflower: 1/2 teaspoon (nervous system support)

Preparation:

1. Combine herbs in a tea strainer
2. Pour 12 oz hot (not boiling) water over herbs
3. Steep covered for 15 minutes
4. Strain and drink warm
5. Add a few drops of stevia if needed for taste

Expected Effects:

- Deep relaxation and stress reduction
- Continued blood purification overnight
- Support for restorative sleep
- Preparation for cellular repair processes

THE SLEEP OPTIMIZATION PROTOCOL

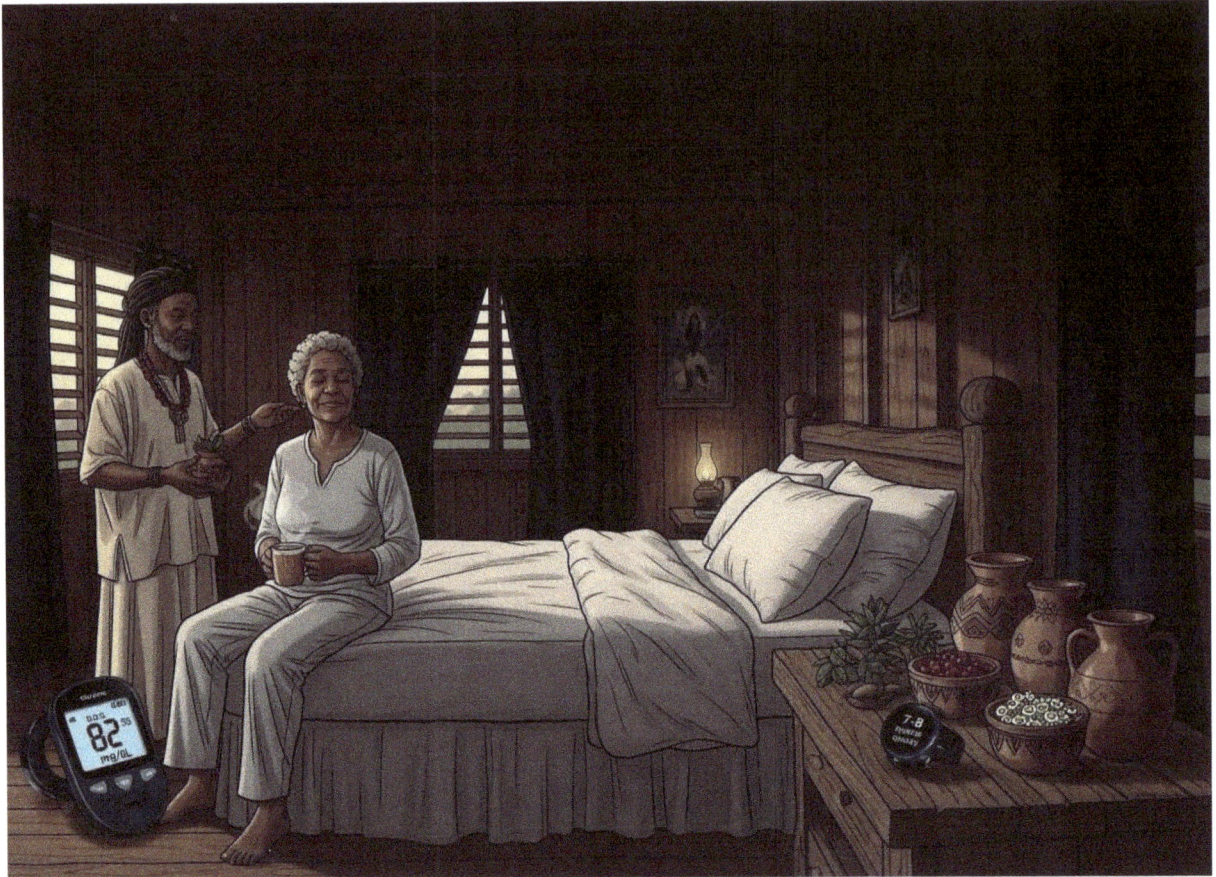

1 Hour Before Bed:

The Sleep and Repair Support Complex:

Ashwagandha - 300mg

- Reduces cortisol levels by 30%
- Promotes deep, restorative sleep
- Supports adrenal recovery overnight
- Improves stress resilience

Melatonin - 1-3mg (start with 1mg)

- Regulates circadian rhythms
- Improves sleep quality and duration
- Provides antioxidant protection
- Supports overnight cellular repair

Alpha-Lipoic Acid - 300mg

- Continuous glucose uptake support overnight
- Provides powerful antioxidant protection during sleep
- Supports nerve regeneration and repair
- Reduces oxidative stress from daily metabolism

30 Minutes Before Bed:

The Final Evening Protocol:

Tart Cherry Extract - 500mg

- Natural source of melatonin
- Reduces inflammation overnight
- Supports deep sleep cycles
- Provides antioxidant protection

Magnesium Glycinate - 200mg (additional dose)

- Promotes muscle relaxation
- Supports a nervous system calm
- Improves sleep quality
- Maintains stable blood sugar overnight

BEDROOM ENVIRONMENT OPTIMIZATION

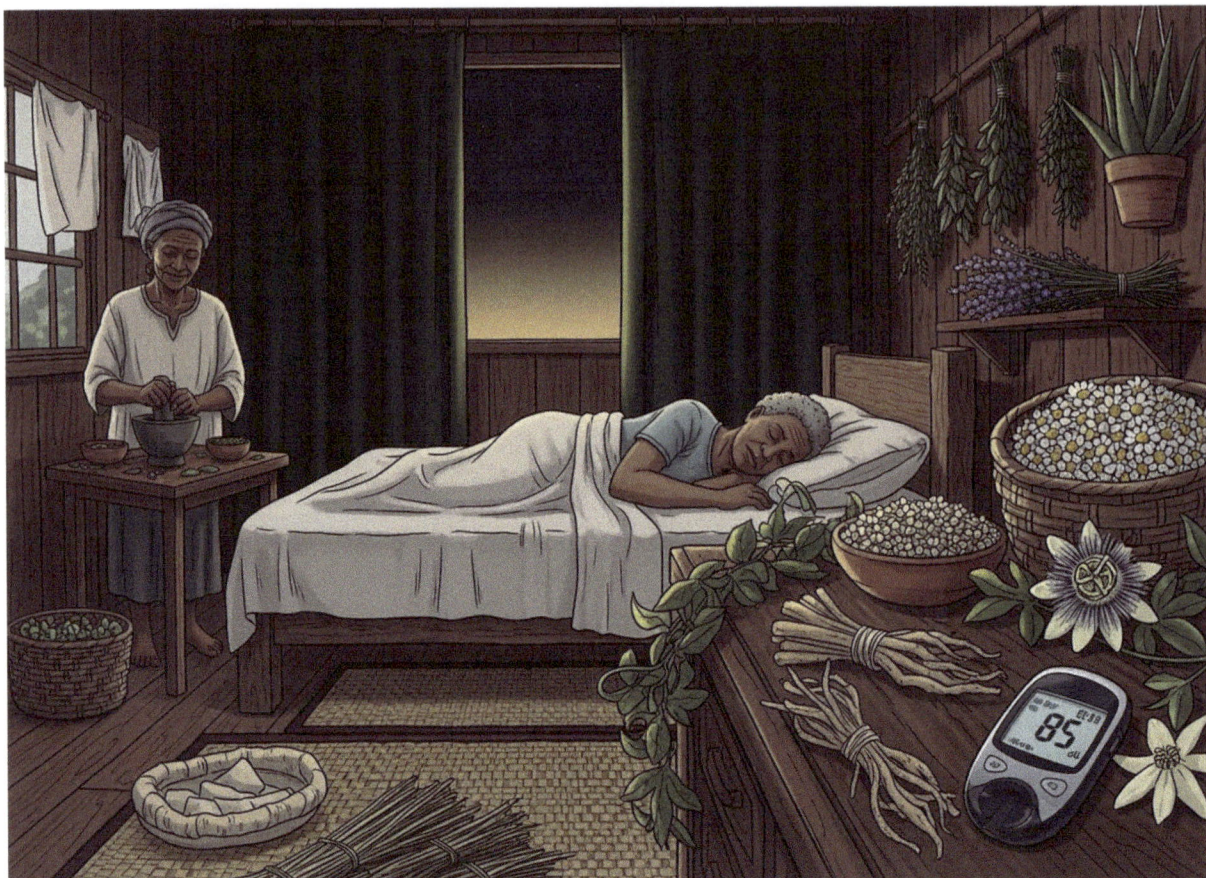

Creating the Healing Sleep Environment:

Temperature Control:

- Keep bedroom between 65-68°F (18-20°C)
- Cool temperatures improve insulin sensitivity
- Supports natural melatonin production
- Promotes deeper sleep phases

Light Management:

- Complete darkness or blackout curtains
- Remove all electronic devices 1 hour before bed
- Use red light bulbs for evening lighting
- Consider a sleep mask if needed

Air Quality:

- Ensure good ventilation
- Consider an air purifier if needed

- Keep humidity between 40-60%
- Remove allergens and irritants

THE OVERNIGHT FASTING PROTOCOL

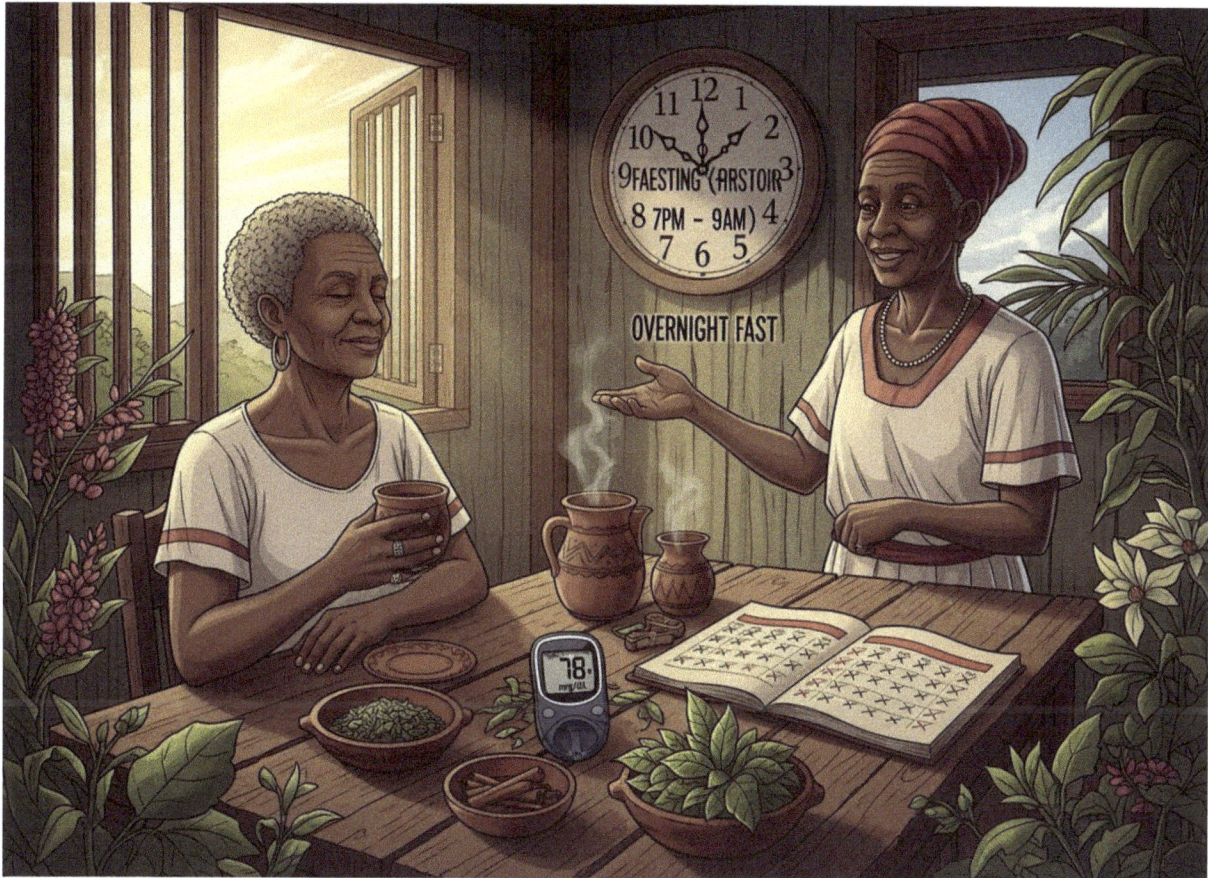

The 12-14 Hour Fast: From your last bite of dinner until your morning lemon water, maintain a complete fast except for:

- Plain water (room temperature preferred)
- Herbal teas without sweeteners
- Emergency glucose tablets only if blood sugar drops dangerously low

Why Overnight Fasting Heals Diabetes:

- Allows insulin levels to drop to baseline
- Improves insulin sensitivity by 25-40%
- Activates cellular autophagy (cellular cleanup)
- Reduces liver glucose production over time
- Promotes fat burning and weight loss

MANAGING OVERNIGHT BLOOD SUGAR

The 3 AM Challenge: Many diabetics experience blood sugar spikes between 2-4 AM due to:

- Dawn phenomenon (natural hormone release)
- Somogyi effect (rebound from overnight lows)
- Stress or poor sleep quality
- Excessive liver glucose production

Prevention Strategies:

- Follow the evening protocol exactly as outlined
- Ensure adequate magnesium intake
- Manage stress with evening relaxation
- Avoid late-night eating or snacking
- Monitor and adjust medications with a doctor

If You Wake Up with High Blood Sugar:

1. Drink 8 oz of water with 1 tablespoon of apple cider vinegar
2. Take 400mg of gymnema sylvestre
3. Do 10 minutes of gentle movement
4. Practice deep breathing exercises
5. Return to bed if possible

SLEEP QUALITY AND DIABETES REVERSAL

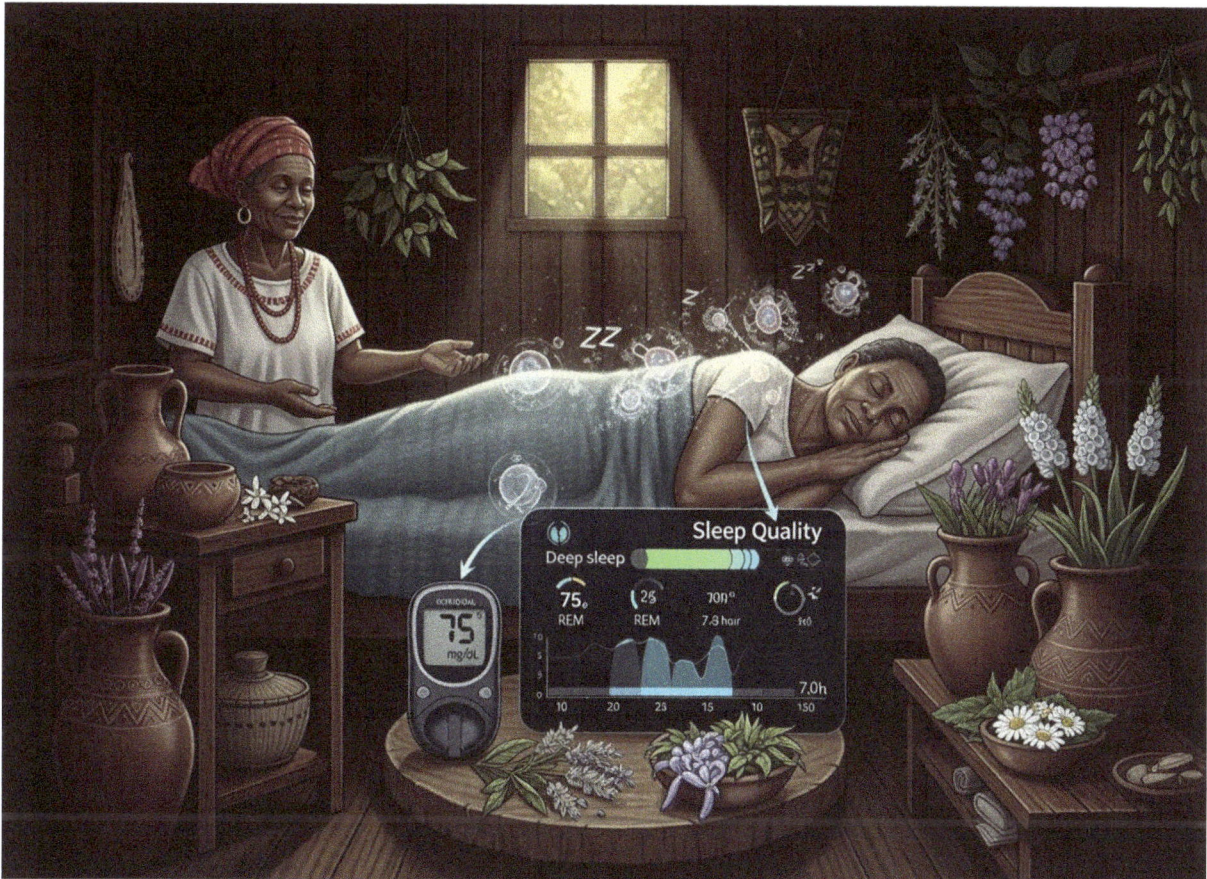

The Sleep-Diabetes Connection: Poor sleep quality directly worsens diabetes through:

- Increased cortisol production
- Reduced insulin sensitivity by 25%
- Increased hunger hormones (ghrelin)
- Decreased satiety hormones (leptin)
- Impaired glucose metabolism

Optimizing Sleep for Healing:

- Aim for 7-9 hours of quality sleep nightly
- Maintain consistent sleep and wake times
- Create a relaxing bedtime routine
- Address sleep disorders (sleep apnea, restless legs)
- Use natural sleep supports rather than medications

TROUBLESHOOTING EVENING CHALLENGES

Problem: Blood sugar spikes after dinner despite supplements. Solutions:

- Take supplements 45 minutes before eating
- Reduce dinner carbohydrates to <10g
- Increase post-meal movement to 30 minutes
- Check for hidden sugars in foods

Problem: Difficulty falling asleep. Solutions:

- Increase magnesium to 600mg total daily
- Add 100mg L-theanine to evening tea
- Practice progressive muscle relaxation
- Ensure complete darkness in the bedroom

Problem: Waking up with high blood sugar. Solutions:

- Eat dinner earlier (4+ hours before bed)
- Add 10mg vanadyl sulfate at bedtime
- Check for sleep apnea or other disorders
- Monitor overnight with a continuous glucose monitor

Problem: Night-time hypoglycemia Solutions:

- Discuss medication timing with the doctor
- Have a small protein snack if blood sugar is <100 at bedtime
- Keep glucose tablets at bedside
- Check for over-medication

THE WEEKLY INTENSIVE EVENING PROTOCOL

Once Per Week (Choose Same Day Each Week):

The Deep Cleanse Evening:

- Extended fasting period (16-18 hours)
- Double dose of blood purification tea
- Epsom salt bath with lavender oil
- Extended meditation or prayer time
- Early bedtime for maximum repair time

Benefits of Weekly Intensive:

- Deeper cellular detoxification
- Enhanced insulin sensitivity reset

- Improved sleep quality
- Accelerated healing and repair
- Stronger connection to the healing process

REAL SUCCESS STORIES

Michael's Sleep Transformation: "I used to wake up at 3 AM with blood sugars over 250. The evening protocol changed everything. Now I sleep through the night and wake up with readings between 90 and 110. The magnesium and evening tea made the biggest difference for me."

Linda's Evening Victory: "Dinner was always my downfall. I'd eat well all day, then blow it with a big dinner and dessert. The evening protocol taught me how to eat lighter at night and actually enjoy it. My overnight readings are now stable, and I wake up refreshed instead of exhausted."

THE EVENING REFLECTION PRACTICE

Before Sleep (5-10 minutes):

Gratitude and Healing Affirmations:

- "I am grateful for my body's ability to heal."
- "Every cell in my body is restoring itself tonight."
- "I wake up tomorrow with renewed health and energy."
- "My blood sugar is stable and balanced."
- "I am free from diabetes and full of vitality."

Daily Progress Review:

- What went well with my protocol today?
- What challenges did I overcome?
- How did I honor my commitment to healing?
- What will I do even better tomorrow?
- How do I feel about my progress?

THE POWER OF EVENING CONSISTENCY

The Compound Effect: Each night, you follow the Evening Restoration Protocol:

- Your insulin sensitivity improves slightly
- Your cellular repair processes become more efficient
- Your sleep quality enhances
- Your morning blood sugars stabilize
- Your overall health transforms

The 30-Day Evening Challenge: Commit to following the complete evening protocol for 30 consecutive days and track:

- Sleep quality scores (1-10 daily)
- Morning blood sugar readings
- Energy levels upon waking
- Overall sense of well-being
- Progress toward diabetes reversal

YOUR PERSONALIZED EVENING STRATEGY

Individual customization may be needed based on:

- Current sleep quality and disorders
- Medication timing and effects
- Work schedule and evening commitments
- Family responsibilities and stress levels

Schedule Your FREE 15-Minute Consultation

During this call, we'll customize your evening protocol to address your specific challenges and ensure optimal overnight healing and blood sugar stability.

THE SACRED EVENING RITUAL

Your evening protocol is more than just a health routine – it's a sacred ritual that honors your body's natural healing wisdom and your commitment to diabetes reversal.

Each evening, as you prepare your restorative tea and take your healing supplements, you participate in a 300-year-old tradition of natural healing and join thousands of others who have found freedom from diabetes.

This ritual represents rest, restoration, and the deep faith that your body heals itself while you sleep.

THE BRIDGE TO TOMORROW

Your evening protocol creates the foundation for tomorrow's success:

Immediate Benefits (during sleep):

- Stable blood sugar throughout the night
- Deep, restorative sleep cycles
- Cellular repair and regeneration
- Stress hormone balance

Morning Benefits:

- Wake up with stable blood sugar
- Natural energy and mental clarity
- Reduced morning medication needs
- Positive momentum for the day

Long-term Benefits (weeks to months):

- Consistent A1C improvements
- Better overall sleep quality
- Reduced diabetes complications
- Complete metabolic transformation

In the next chapter, we'll explore the foods that heal versus those that harm – the nutritional foundation that supports or sabotages your diabetes reversal journey.

CHAPTER 10
THE ALLOWED FOODS THAT HEAL

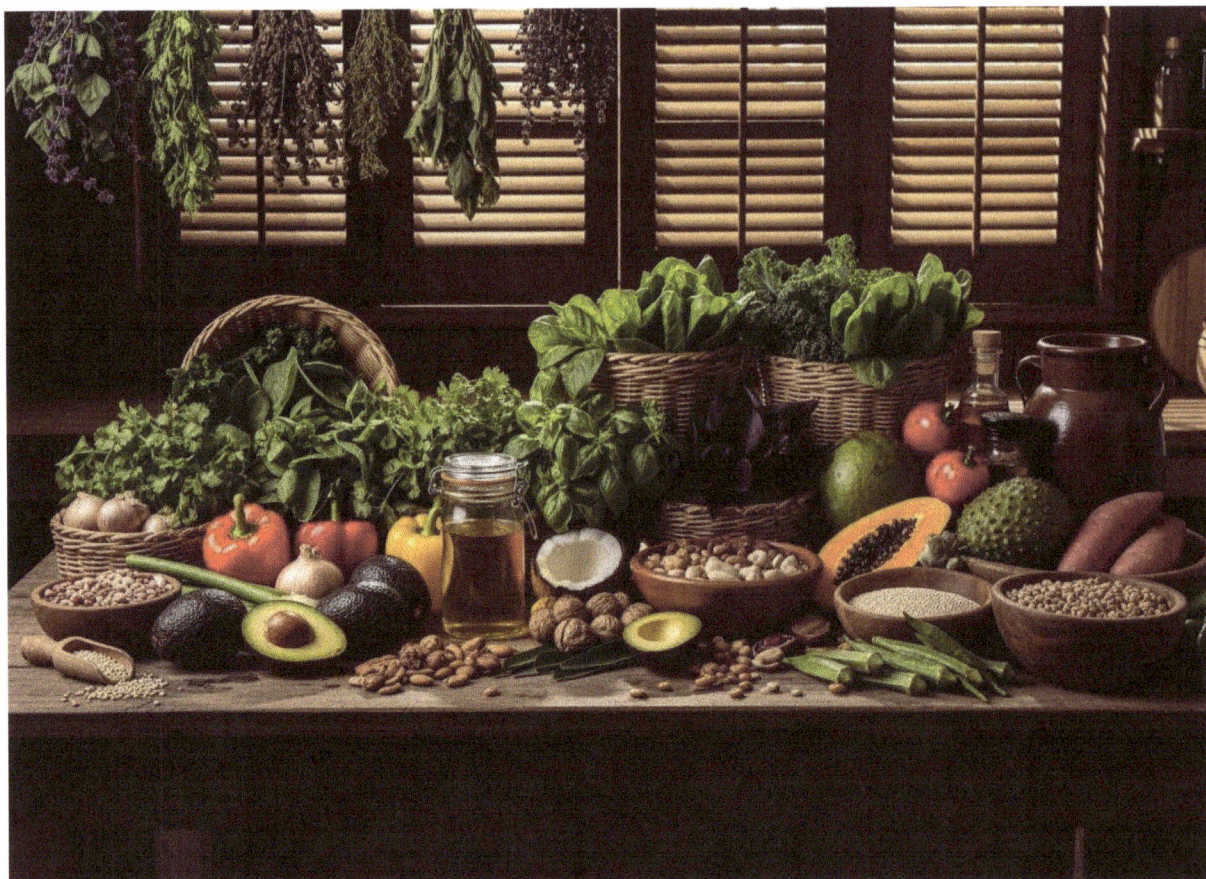

"Food is either medicine or poison. There is no neutral ground when it comes to diabetes reversal. Every bite either moves you toward healing or away from it."

After 300 years of traditional healing and working with thousands of diabetics, one truth has become crystal clear: the foods you eat are either actively healing your diabetes or actively making it worse.

There are no "neutral" foods for diabetics. Every meal is an opportunity to either support your body's natural healing mechanisms or to sabotage your progress with blood sugar spikes, inflammation, and metabolic dysfunction.

This chapter will transform how you think about food – not as mere calories or macronutrients, but as powerful medicine that can reverse diabetes when chosen correctly.

THE HEALING FOOD PHILOSOPHY

Food as Medicine My Maroon ancestors understood that food and medicine were inseparable. The same plants that healed disease also nourished the body. This wasn't convenience – it was wisdom.

Modern nutrition has lost this connection, treating food as fuel rather than medicine. But for diabetes reversal, we must return to the ancient understanding that every meal is an opportunity for healing.

The Three Categories of Food:

1. **Healing Foods** - Actively reverse diabetes and restore metabolic health
2. **Neutral Foods** - Neither help nor harm (very few foods fall into this category)
3. **Harmful Foods** - Worsen diabetes, increase inflammation, and prevent healing

THE METABOLIC HEALING HIERARCHY

TIER 1: SUPER HEALING FOODS These foods actively reverse diabetes through multiple mechanisms:

Leafy Green Vegetables

- Spinach, kale, arugula, Swiss chard, collard greens
- **Healing Mechanisms:** High in magnesium for insulin sensitivity, rich in antioxidants, virtually no carbohydrates
- **Daily Target:** 2-3 cups raw or 1-2 cups cooked
- **Best Preparation:** Raw in salads, lightly sautéed, steamed, or in green smoothies

Cruciferous Vegetables

- Broccoli, cauliflower, Brussels sprouts, cabbage, bok choy
- **Healing Mechanisms:** Contain sulforaphane, which improves insulin sensitivity, and high fiber slows glucose absorption
- **Daily Target:** 1-2 cups daily
- **Best Preparation:** Lightly steamed, roasted, or raw

Wild-Caught Fatty Fish

- Salmon, sardines, mackerel, anchovies, herring
- **Healing Mechanisms:** Omega-3 fatty acids reduce inflammation, and high-quality protein stabilizes blood sugar
- **Weekly Target:** 3-4 servings
- **Best Preparation:** Grilled, baked, or poached with herbs and lemon

Avocados

- **Healing Mechanisms:** Monounsaturated fats improve insulin sensitivity, fiber slows glucose absorption, and potassium supports cellular function
- **Daily Target:** 1/2 to 1 whole avocado
- **Best Uses:** Raw in salads, as guacamole, or blended in smoothies

Raw Nuts and Seeds

- Almonds, walnuts, pecans, pumpkin seeds, chia seeds, flaxseeds
- **Healing Mechanisms:** Healthy fats stabilize blood sugar, magnesium improves insulin function, and protein provides satiety
- **Daily Target:** 1/4 cup (about 1 ounce)
- **Best Preparation:** Raw, unsalted, soaked overnight for better digestion

TIER 2: STRONG HEALING FOODS

Organic Eggs

- **Healing Mechanisms:** Complete protein stabilizes blood sugar, choline supports liver function, and healthy fats provide satiety
- **Daily Target:** 2-3 whole eggs
- **Best Preparation:** Soft-boiled, poached, or scrambled in coconut oil

Grass-Fed Meat and Poultry

- Beef, lamb, chicken, turkey (grass-fed/pasture-raised only)
- **Healing Mechanisms:** High-quality protein stabilizes blood sugar, B-vitamins support metabolism, no carbohydrates
- **Daily Target:** 4-6 oz per meal
- **Best Preparation:** Grilled, roasted, or slow-cooked with herbs

Coconut Products

- Coconut oil, coconut milk, unsweetened coconut flakes
- **Healing Mechanisms:** Medium-chain triglycerides provide stable energy, and lauric acid has antimicrobial properties
- **Daily Target:** 1-2 tablespoons coconut oil, 1/4 cup coconut milk
- **Best Uses:** Cooking oil, coffee additive, smoothie ingredient

Herbs and Spices

- Turmeric, ginger, cinnamon, garlic, oregano, basil, rosemary
- **Healing Mechanisms:** Powerful anti-inflammatory compounds, many directly improve insulin sensitivity
- **Daily Target:** Use liberally in all meals

- **Best Preparation:** Fresh when possible, dried herbs and spices in cooking

Low-Glycemic Vegetables

- Asparagus, zucchini, bell peppers, cucumber, radishes, celery
- **Healing Mechanisms:** High fiber, low carbohydrates, rich in nutrients and antioxidants
- **Daily Target:** 3-4 cups daily
- **Best Preparation:** Raw, steamed, roasted, or sautéed

The Perfect Diabetic Meal Structure:

- **50% Non-starchy vegetables** (variety of colors and textures)
- **25% Quality protein** (animal or plant-based)
- **25% Healthy fats** (avocado, nuts, seeds, oils)
- **0% Grains, starches, or sugars**

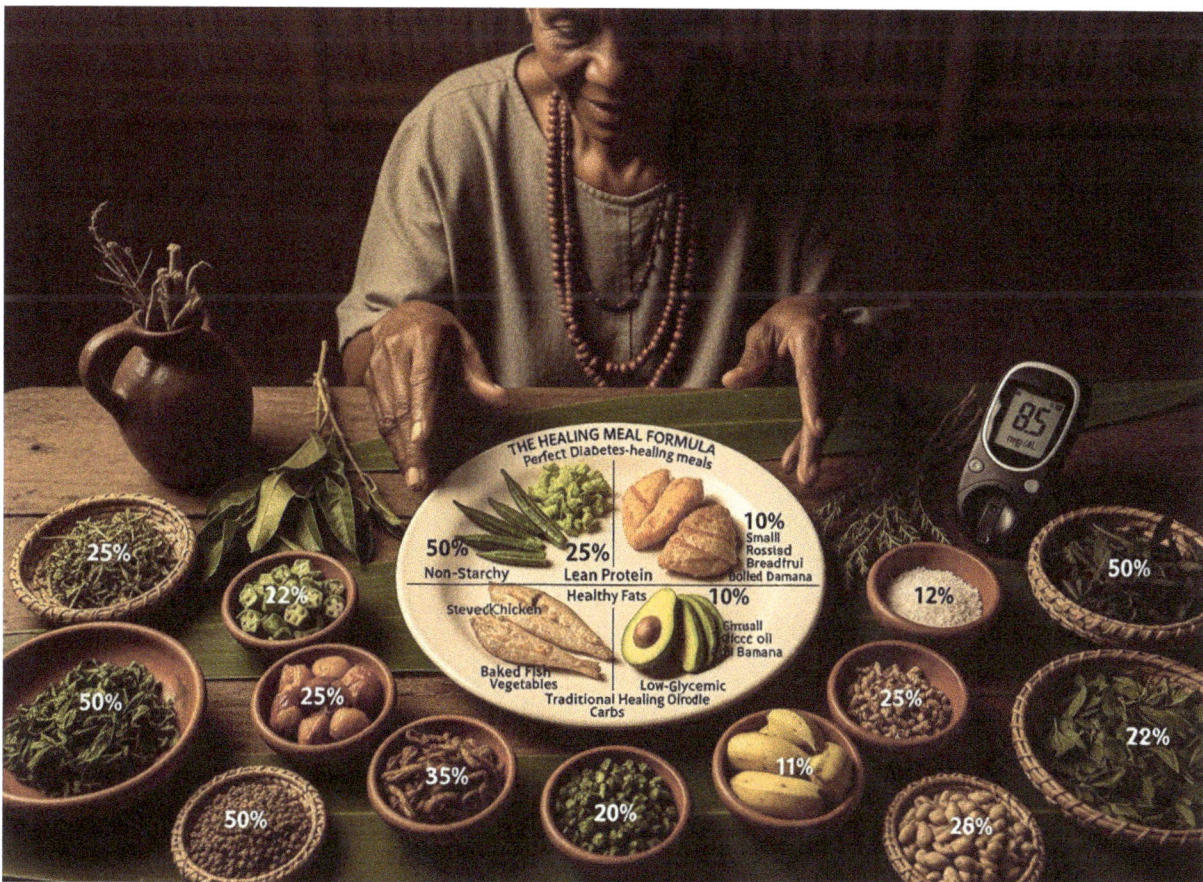

Sample Healing Meals:

Breakfast: The Metabolic Reset Bowl

- 2 cups baby spinach and arugula
- 2 scrambled eggs cooked in coconut oil

- 1/2 avocado sliced
- 2 tablespoons pumpkin seeds
- 1 tablespoon olive oil drizzle
- Fresh herbs and lemon juice

Lunch: The Power Salad

- 3 cups mixed greens (kale, spinach, arugula)
- 4 oz grilled wild salmon
- 1/4 cup raw walnuts
- 1/2 cucumber diced
- 2 tablespoons avocado oil dressing
- Fresh dill and lemon

Dinner: The Healing Plate

- 6 oz grass-fed beef or lamb
- 2 cups roasted broccoli and cauliflower
- Large mixed green salad
- 2 tablespoons olive oil and herbs
- Sautéed garlic and onions

HEALING BEVERAGES

TIER 1: SUPER HEALING DRINKS

Pure Water

- **Target:** Half your body weight in ounces daily
- **Best Types:** Filtered, spring, or reverse osmosis
- **Enhancements:** Add lemon, cucumber, or mint

Herbal Teas

- Green tea, white tea, oolong tea, and herbal blends
- **Benefits:** Antioxidants, improved insulin sensitivity, hydration without calories
- **Daily Target:** 2-4 cups
- **Best Choices:** Organic, loose-leaf when possible

Bone Broth

- **Benefits:** Collagen for gut healing, minerals for cellular function, protein for satiety
- **Daily Target:** 1-2 cups
- **Best Preparation:** Homemade from grass-fed bones, slow-cooked 24+ hours

TIER 2: HEALING DRINKS

Coconut Water (unsweetened)

- **Benefits:** Natural electrolytes, lower in sugar than fruit juices
- **Limit:** 4-6 oz daily maximum
- **Best Use:** Post-exercise hydration

Vegetable Juices (low-sodium)

- **Benefits:** Concentrated nutrients, minimal sugar impact
- **Best Choices:** Celery, cucumber, leafy greens, herbs
- **Limit:** 4-6 oz daily

HEALING FATS AND OILS

TIER 1: SUPER HEALING FATS

Extra Virgin Olive Oil

- **Benefits:** Monounsaturated fats improve insulin sensitivity, and antioxidants reduce inflammation
- **Daily Target:** 2-3 tablespoons
- **Best Uses:** Salad dressings, low-heat cooking, finishing oil

Coconut Oil

- **Benefits:** Medium-chain triglycerides provide stable energy, antimicrobial properties, and support thyroid function
- **Daily Target:** 1-2 tablespoons
- **Best Uses:** High-heat cooking, coffee additive, baking substitute

Avocado Oil

- **Benefits:** High smoke point for cooking, monounsaturated fats, and vitamin E
- **Daily Target:** 1-2 tablespoons
- **Best Uses:** High-heat cooking, salad dressings, mayonnaise base

Raw Nuts and Seed Oils

- Walnut oil, flaxseed oil, hemp seed oil (cold-pressed only)
- **Benefits:** Omega-3 fatty acids, anti-inflammatory compounds
- **Daily Target:** 1 tablespoon
- **Best Uses:** Salad dressings, smoothies, finishing oils (never heated)

TIER 2: HEALING FATS

Grass-Fed Butter

- **Benefits:** Conjugated linoleic acid (CLA), vitamin K2, butyric acid for gut health
- **Daily Target:** 1-2 tablespoons
- **Best Uses:** Low-heat cooking, spreading, coffee additive

Ghee (Clarified Butter)

- **Benefits:** High smoke point, lactose-free, rich in fat-soluble vitamins
- **Daily Target:** 1-2 tablespoons
- **Best Uses:** High-heat cooking, Indian cuisine, Ayurvedic preparations

HEALING PROTEINS

TIER 1: SUPER HEALING PROTEINS

Wild-Caught Fish

- Salmon, sardines, mackerel, anchovies, cod, halibut
- **Benefits:** Complete amino acids, omega-3 fatty acids, low mercury
- **Daily Target:** 4-6 oz per serving
- **Best Preparation:** Grilled, baked, or poached with herbs and lemon

Pasture-Raised Eggs

- **Benefits:** Complete protein, choline for liver health, healthy fats
- **Daily Target:** 2-3 whole eggs
- **Best Preparation:** Soft-boiled, poached, scrambled in healthy fats

Grass-Fed Beef and Lamb

- **Benefits:** Complete amino acids, CLA, iron, B-vitamins
- **Daily Target:** 4-6 oz per serving
- **Best Preparation:** Grilled, roasted, slow-cooked with vegetables

TIER 2: HEALING PROTEINS

Organic Poultry

- Chicken, turkey, duck (pasture-raised preferred)
- **Benefits:** Lean protein, B-vitamins, selenium
- **Daily Target:** 4-6 oz per serving
- **Best Preparation:** Roasted, grilled, slow-cooked with herbs

Plant-Based Proteins

- Hemp seeds, chia seeds, spirulina, chlorella
- **Benefits:** Complete amino acids, minerals, antioxidants

- **Daily Target:** 2-3 tablespoons of seeds, 1 teaspoon algae
- **Best Uses:** Smoothies, salads, protein powders

HEALING SEASONINGS AND FLAVOR ENHANCERS

TIER 1: SUPER HEALING SEASONINGS

Ceylon Cinnamon

- **Benefits:** Improves insulin sensitivity by 40%, mimics insulin action
- **Daily Target:** 1/2 to 1 teaspoon
- **Best Uses:** Teas, smoothies, meat rubs, vegetable seasonings

Turmeric with Black Pepper

- **Benefits:** Powerful anti-inflammatory, improves insulin sensitivity
- **Daily Target:** 1/2 teaspoon turmeric with a pinch of black pepper
- **Best Uses:** Curries, golden milk, roasted vegetables, meat marinades

Fresh Ginger

- **Benefits:** Improves insulin sensitivity, aids digestion, anti-inflammatory
- **Daily Target:** 1-2 teaspoons fresh grated or 1/2 teaspoon dried
- **Best Uses:** Teas, stir-fries, marinades, fresh juices

Garlic

- **Benefits:** Improves insulin sensitivity, antimicrobial, and cardiovascular support
- **Daily Target:** 2-3 cloves fresh or 1/2 teaspoon powder
- **Best Uses:** Roasted, sautéed, raw in dressings, marinades

TIER 2: HEALING SEASONINGS

Fresh Herbs

- Basil, oregano, thyme, rosemary, cilantro, parsley
- **Benefits:** Antioxidants, anti-inflammatory compounds, digestive support
- **Daily Target:** Use liberally
- **Best Uses:** Fresh in salads, dried in cooking, and herb-infused oils

Celtic Sea Salt and Himalayan Salt

- **Benefits:** Essential minerals, electrolyte balance, supports adrenal function

- **Daily Target:** 1/2 to 1 teaspoon total daily
- **Best Uses:** Cooking, seasoning, sole water for hydration

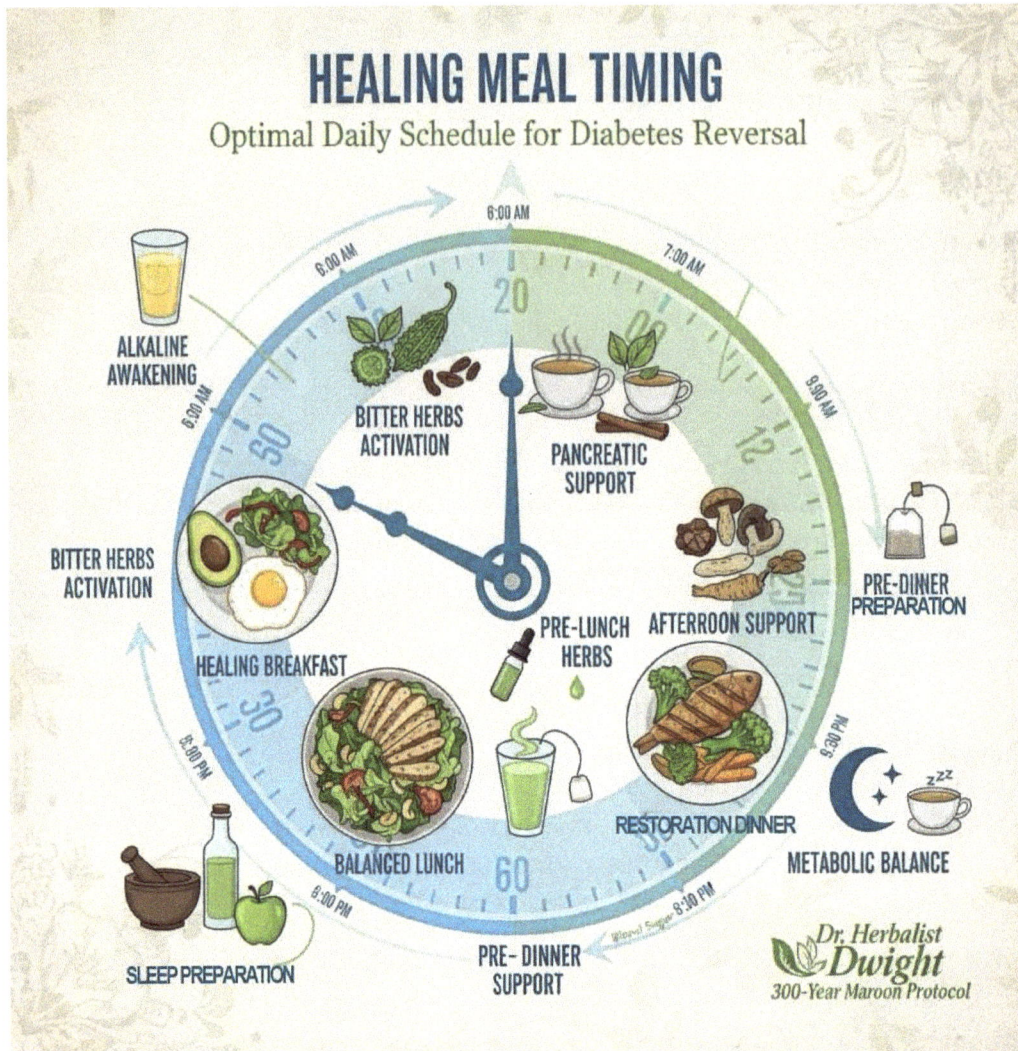

HEALING MEAL TIMING
Optimal Daily Schedule for Diabetes Reversal

The Optimal Eating Schedule:

Morning (7-9 AM):

- Break overnight fast with healing foods
- Emphasize protein and healthy fats
- Include bitter herbs and vegetables

Midday (12-2 PM):

- The largest meal is when the digestive fire is strongest
- Balance of all macronutrients
- Include a variety of healing vegetables

Evening (5-7 PM):

- Lighter meal, easier to digest
- Emphasize vegetables and moderate protein
- Finish eating 3-4 hours before bed

Intermittent Fasting Windows:

- 12-14 hours overnight (dinner to breakfast)
- 16-18 hours once weekly for deeper healing
- Listen to your body's hunger and satiety signals

FOOD COMBINING FOR OPTIMAL HEALING

Synergistic Combinations:

Turmeric + Black Pepper + Healthy Fat

- Increases curcumin absorption by 2000%
- Best combination: Golden milk with coconut oil

Iron-Rich Foods + Vitamin C

- Improves iron absorption for energy and metabolism
- Best combination: Spinach salad with lemon dressing

Healthy Fats + Fat-Soluble Vitamins

- Maximizes absorption of vitamins A, D, E, and K
- Best combination: Avocado with leafy greens

Protein + Chromium-Rich Foods

- Improves insulin sensitivity and glucose metabolism
- Best combination: Eggs with nutritional yeast

HEALING FOOD PREPARATION METHODS

TIER 1: SUPER HEALING METHODS

Raw Preparation

- **Benefits:** Preserves enzymes, maximizes nutrient content, easiest digestion
- **Best For:** Leafy greens, nuts, seeds, herbs, and some vegetables
- **Daily Target:** 50% of vegetables consumed raw

Light Steaming

- **Benefits:** Preserves nutrients while improving digestibility
- **Best For:** Cruciferous vegetables, asparagus, green beans
- **Method:** Steam 3-5 minutes until bright colored and tender-crisp

Low-Temperature Roasting

- **Benefits:** Concentrates flavors while preserving nutrients
- **Best For:** Root vegetables, Brussels sprouts, cauliflower
- **Method:** 350°F or lower, with healthy oils and herbs

TIER 2: HEALING METHODS

Sautéing in Healthy Fats

- **Benefits:** Quick cooking preserves nutrients, adds healthy fats
- **Best For:** Leafy greens, mushrooms, onions, garlic
- **Method:** Medium heat, coconut oil or ghee, 2-3 minutes

Slow Cooking

- **Benefits:** Breaks down tough fibers, concentrates flavors, convenient
- **Best For:** Tough cuts of meat, bone broths, stews
- **Method:** Low heat, 4-8 hours, with healing herbs and vegetables

HEALING FOOD SOURCING

Quality Priorities:

Tier 1: Essential Organic

- Leafy greens (high pesticide residue)
- Berries (thin skin absorbs chemicals)
- Animal products (concentrate toxins)

Tier 2: Preferred Organic

- All vegetables, when the budget allows
- Nuts and seeds
- Herbs and spices

Sourcing Guidelines:

- Local farmers' markets for the freshest produce
- Community-supported agriculture (CSA) programs
- Grass-fed/pasture-raised animal products
- Wild-caught fish from reputable sources

- Organic when possible, conventional when necessary

MEAL PREP FOR HEALING SUCCESS

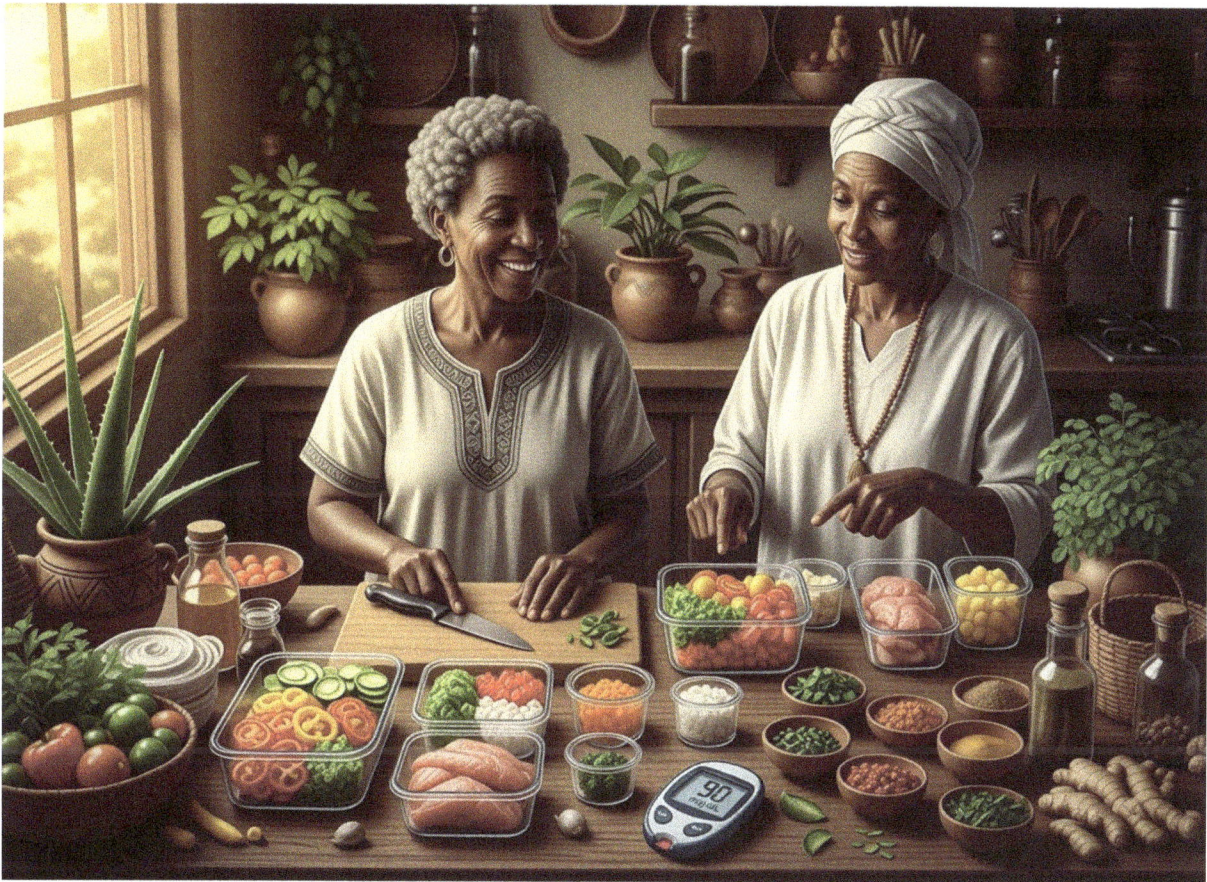

Weekly Preparation Strategy:

Sunday Prep Session (2-3 hours):

- Wash and chop all vegetables for the week
- Cook proteins in bulk (roasted chicken, hard-boiled eggs)
- Prepare healing dressings and sauces
- Make bone broth in a slow cooker
- Portion nuts and seeds into daily servings

Daily Fresh Additions:

- Fresh herbs and microgreens
- Avocado (cut fresh daily)
- Fresh lemon juice
- Delicate greens that don't store well

HEALING FOOD COMBINATIONS FOR SPECIFIC BENEFITS

For Blood Sugar Stability:

- Protein + healthy fat + non-starchy vegetables
- Example: Salmon + avocado + spinach salad

For Inflammation Reduction:

- Omega-3 rich foods + antioxidant vegetables + anti-inflammatory spices
- Example: Sardines + kale + turmeric dressing

For Insulin Sensitivity:

- Chromium-rich foods + magnesium-rich foods + cinnamon
- Example: Eggs + spinach + cinnamon tea

For Cellular Repair:

- Antioxidant-rich vegetables + quality protein + healing herbs
- Example: Colorful vegetable stir-fry + grass-fed beef + fresh herbs

TRACKING YOUR HEALING FOODS

Daily Food Log:

- Record all foods consumed
- Note blood sugar responses
- Track energy levels and mood
- Identify personal trigger foods

Weekly Assessment:

- Percentage of healing foods consumed
- A variety of vegetables included
- Quality of protein sources
- Balance of healthy fats

Monthly Evaluation:

- Overall dietary improvements
- Blood sugar stability patterns
- Weight and body composition changes
- Energy and vitality levels

REAL SUCCESS STORIES

Patricia's Food Transformation: "I thought I was eating healthy with my whole grain cereals and low-fat yogurt. When I switched to the healing foods protocol - eggs for breakfast, big salads for lunch, and grass-fed meat with vegetables for dinner - my blood sugars dropped 50 points within two weeks. The food actually tastes better than what I was eating before!"

Robert's Meal Prep Success: "The meal prep strategy changed everything for me. Spending Sunday afternoon preparing healing foods for the week meant I never had to make decisions when I was hungry and tempted. My A1C dropped from 8.9 to 5.8 in four months just by consistently eating healing foods."

YOUR PERSONALIZED HEALING FOOD PLAN

Individual customization may be needed based on:

- Food allergies and sensitivities
- Cultural and family food preferences
- Budget and accessibility constraints
- Cooking skills and time availability

[Schedule Your FREE 15-Minute Consultation](#)

During this call, we'll create a personalized healing food plan that fits your lifestyle, preferences, and specific health needs.

THE HEALING FOOD COMMITMENT

Choosing healing foods is more than just a dietary change – it's a commitment to honoring your body's natural healing capacity and providing it with the tools it needs to manage diabetes effectively.

Every meal becomes an opportunity to either support or sabotage your healing journey. When you consistently choose foods that heal, you're not just managing diabetes – you're actively reversing it.

In the next chapter, we'll explore the foods that harm – the dietary saboteurs that must be eliminated for complete diabetes reversal.

CHAPTER 11
FOODS TO AVOID AND WHY

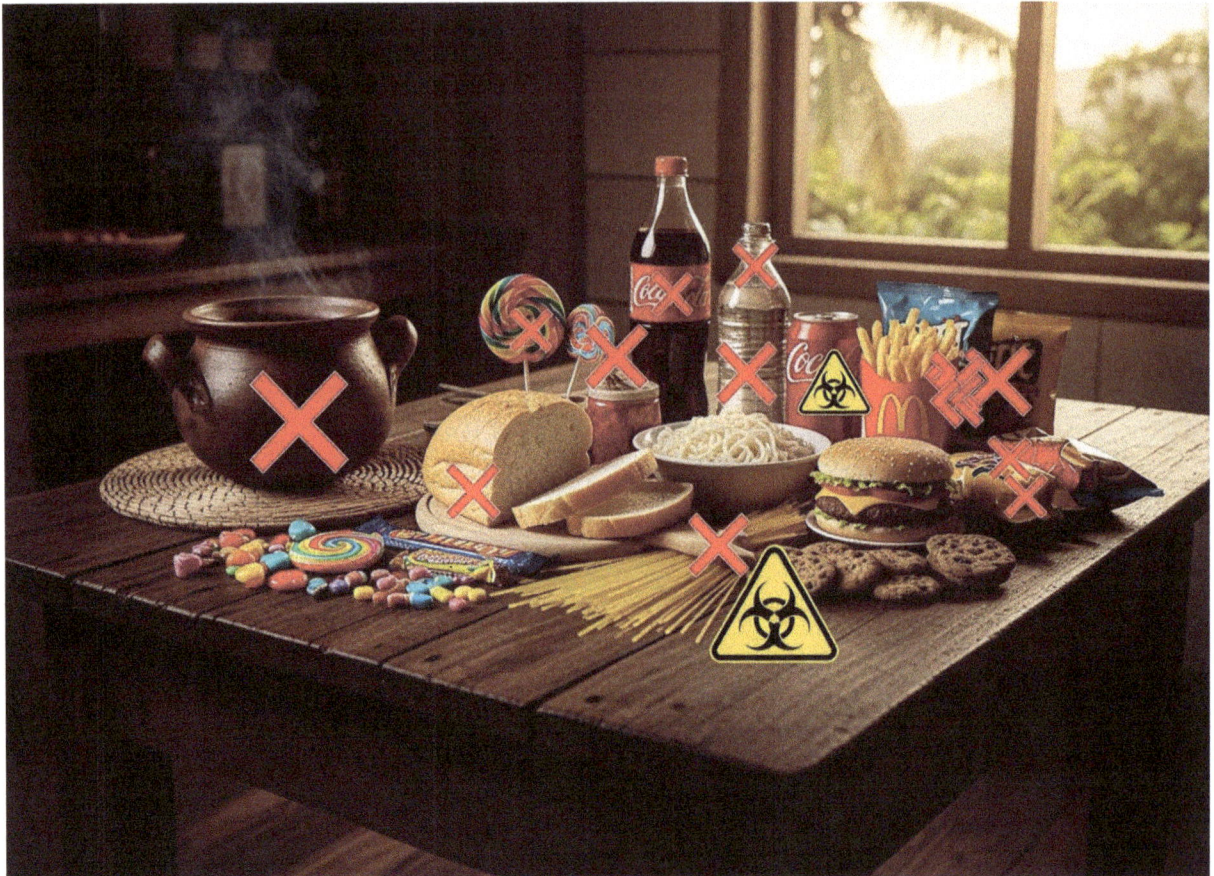

"The foods that created your diabetes cannot heal your diabetes. To reverse this condition, you must eliminate the dietary saboteurs that keep you trapped in metabolic dysfunction."

This may be the most important chapter in this book. While healing foods actively reverse diabetes, harmful foods actively worsen it – often within minutes of consumption.

After working with thousands of diabetics over 65 years, I've seen the same pattern repeatedly: those who eliminate harmful foods completely achieve diabetes reversal, while those who continue eating them in "moderation" remain trapped in medication dependence.

There is no middle ground. There are no "cheat days" when it comes to diabetes reversal. Every harmful food you consume is a step backward on your healing journey.

THE METABOLIC POISON PRINCIPLE

Why "Everything in Moderation" Fails for Diabetics

The conventional advice of "everything in moderation" is metabolic poison for diabetics. Your body is already in a state of metabolic dysfunction – it cannot process certain foods as efficiently as a healthy person can.

Telling a diabetic they can eat sugar "in moderation" is like telling an alcoholic they can drink "in moderation." The underlying metabolic dysfunction makes moderation impossible.

The Inflammatory Cascade

Harmful foods trigger an inflammatory cascade that:

- Worsens insulin resistance within hours
- Damages pancreatic beta cells
- Increases oxidative stress throughout the body
- Disrupts gut bacteria balance
- Elevates stress hormones
- Sabotages sleep quality

One "moderate" serving of the wrong food can undo weeks of progress.

TIER 1: THE METABOLIC DESTROYERS

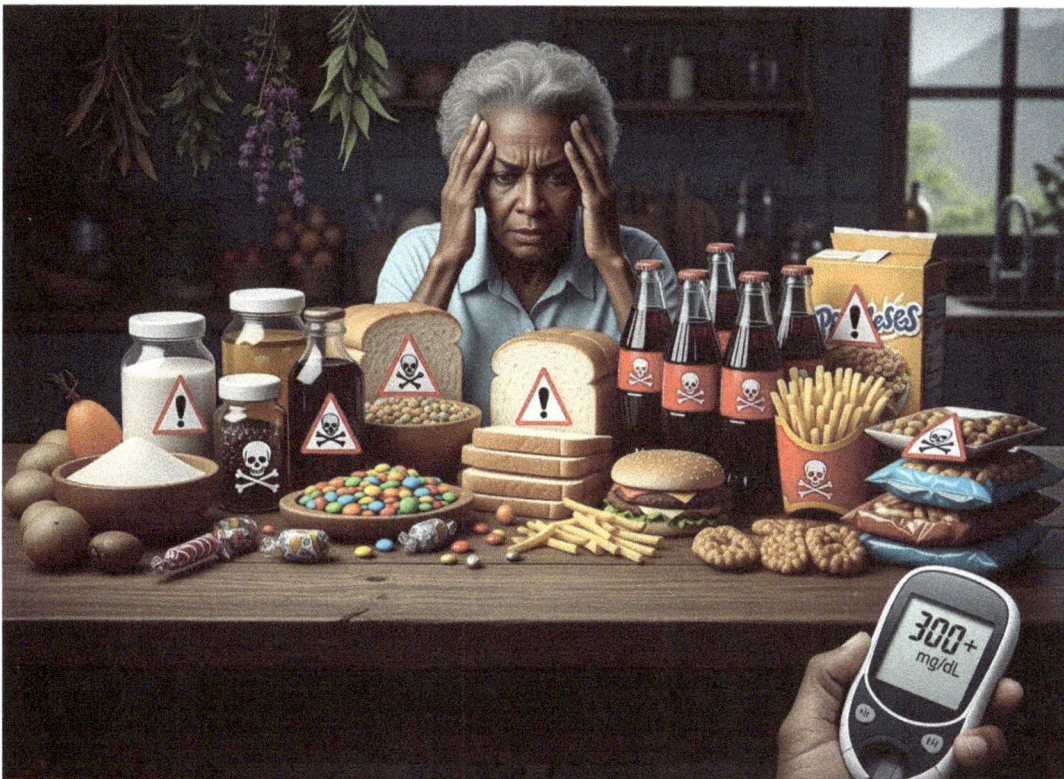

These foods cause immediate and severe metabolic damage. They must be eliminated completely and permanently.

REFINED SUGARS AND SWEETENERS

White Sugar, Brown Sugar, Raw Sugar

- **Why They're Toxic:** Cause immediate blood sugar spikes to 300+ mg/dL, trigger massive insulin release, create addiction-like cravings
- **Hidden Sources:** Condiments, salad dressings, marinades, processed foods, medications
- **Blood Sugar Impact:** 50-100 point spike within 30 minutes
- **Metabolic Damage:** Glycates proteins, damages blood vessels, and exhausts the pancreas

High Fructose Corn Syrup

- **Why It's Worse Than Sugar:** Bypasses normal glucose regulation, is directly converted to fat by the liver, more addictive than cocaine
- **Hidden Sources:** Sodas, fruit juices, processed foods, condiments, bread
- **Blood Sugar Impact:** Delayed but severe spike, followed by a crash
- **Metabolic Damage:** Causes fatty liver, increases insulin resistance, triggers inflammation

Artificial Sweeteners

- **The Deception:** Marketed as "diabetic-friendly" but actually worsens diabetes
- **Types to Avoid:** Aspartame, sucralose, saccharin, acesulfame potassium
- **Why They're Harmful:** Disrupt gut bacteria, increase glucose intolerance, trigger insulin response despite no calories
- **Hidden Sources:** Diet sodas, sugar-free products, medications, protein powders

Agave Nectar and "Natural" Sweeteners

- **The Marketing Lie:** Promoted as healthy alternatives but often worse than sugar
- **Why They're Harmful:** Higher fructose content than high fructose corn syrup
- **Blood Sugar Impact:** Severe delayed spike, crashes, cravings
- **Metabolic Damage:** Rapid development of fatty liver, insulin resistance

REFINED GRAINS AND STARCHES

White Bread, Bagels, Rolls

- **Why They're Toxic:** Convert to glucose faster than table sugar, causing severe blood sugar spikes
- **Blood Sugar Impact:** 100-150 point spike within 45 minutes

- **Metabolic Damage:** Triggers insulin resistance, promotes fat storage, causes inflammation
- **No Safe Amount:** Even one slice can derail progress for days

Pasta (All Types)

- **The Whole Grain Lie:** Whole-grain pasta is only marginally better than white pasta
- **Blood Sugar Impact:** Sustained elevation for 3-4 hours
- **Metabolic Damage:** Keeps insulin elevated, prevents fat burning, worsens insulin resistance
- **Hidden Sources:** Salads, soups, casseroles, "healthy" frozen meals

Rice (White and Brown)

- **Why Brown Rice Isn't Better:** Still causes significant blood sugar elevation
- **Blood Sugar Impact:** 80-120 point spike, sustained elevation
- **Metabolic Damage:** Promotes insulin resistance, prevents ketosis, feeds harmful gut bacteria
- **Cultural Challenge:** Often considered a "healthy" staple food

Breakfast Cereals

- **The Marketing Deception:** Even "healthy" cereals cause severe blood sugar spikes
- **Types to Avoid:** All cereals, including granola, muesli, oatmeal
- **Blood Sugar Impact:** 150+ point spike, followed by a crash and cravings
- **Metabolic Damage:** Sets up the entire day for blood sugar instability

Crackers and Chips

- **Why They're Worse Than Candy:** Often cause higher blood sugar spikes than pure sugar
- **Types to Avoid:** All crackers, potato chips, corn chips, rice cakes
- **Blood Sugar Impact:** Rapid spike, sustained elevation for hours
- **Hidden Dangers:** High in inflammatory oils, preservatives, and artificial flavors

PROCESSED AND PACKAGED FOODS

Frozen Meals and TV Dinners

- **The Convenience Trap:** Loaded with hidden sugars, starches, and preservatives
- **Why They're Harmful:** Designed for shelf-life, not health; contain multiple blood sugar spiking ingredients
- **Hidden Sugars:** Often 15-30g of added sugars per meal
- **Metabolic Impact:** Unpredictable blood sugar responses, inflammation, nutrient deficiencies

Canned Soups and Sauces

- **The Sodium-Sugar Double Hit:** High in both blood pressure-raising sodium and blood sugar-spiking sugars
- **Hidden Sources:** Tomato sauce, pasta sauce, salad dressings, marinades
- **Blood Sugar Impact:** Often overlooked but a significant contributor to spikes
- **Better Alternatives:** Homemade versions with fresh ingredients

Processed Meats

- **Types to Avoid:** Hot dogs, deli meats, sausages, bacon (conventional)
- **Why They're Harmful:** Nitrates, preservatives, hidden sugars, inflammatory oils
- **Blood Sugar Impact:** Moderate but sustained elevation
- **Cancer Risk:** Classified as Group 1 carcinogens by WHO

TIER 2: THE INFLAMMATORY ACCELERATORS

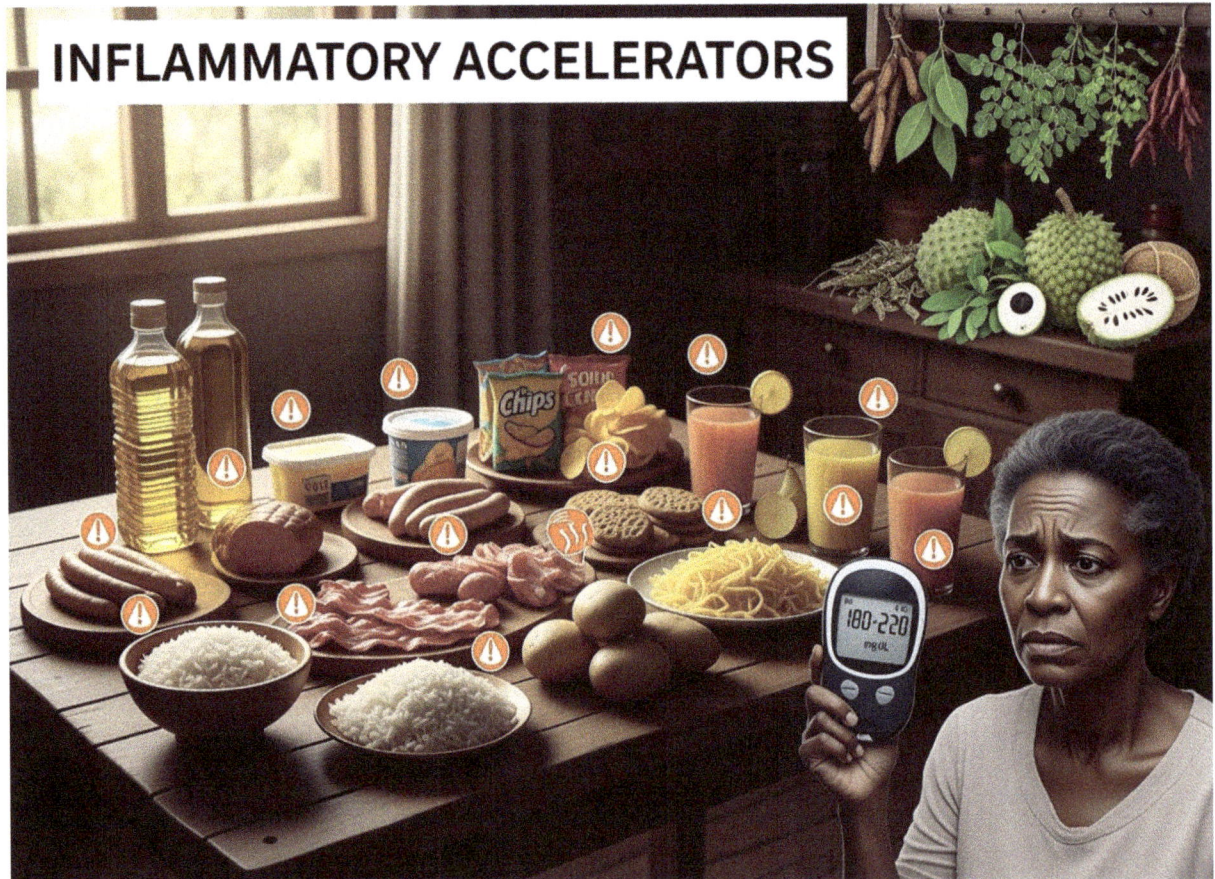

These foods may not spike blood sugar as dramatically, but create systemic inflammation that worsens insulin resistance over time.

INDUSTRIAL SEED OILS

Vegetable Oils

- **Types to Avoid:** Soybean, corn, canola, cottonseed, safflower, sunflower oils
- **Why They're Toxic:** High in omega-6 fatty acids, they promote inflammation, and oxidize easily when heated
- **Hidden Sources:** Restaurant foods, processed foods, salad dressings, and mayonnaise
- **Metabolic Damage:** Worsens insulin resistance, increase oxidative stress, disrupts cellular membranes

Margarine and Fake Butter

- **The Trans Fat Disaster:** Even "trans-fat-free" versions contain harmful industrial oils
- **Why They're Harmful:** Interfere with insulin signaling, promote inflammation, disrupt hormone production
- **Blood Sugar Impact:** Indirect but significant worsening of insulin resistance
- **Better Alternative:** Grass-fed butter, ghee, or coconut oil

DAIRY PRODUCTS (CONVENTIONAL)

Milk (All Types)

- **The Lactose Problem:** Milk sugar (lactose) causes blood sugar spikes in many adults
- **Hidden Sugars:** Even unsweetened milk contains 12g of natural sugars per cup
- **Blood Sugar Impact:** 30-50 point spike, varies by individual
- **Inflammatory Response:** Casein protein triggers inflammation in sensitive individuals

Yogurt (Conventional)

- **The Probiotic Myth:** Most commercial yogurts are loaded with added sugars
- **Sugar Content:** Often 20-30g sugar per serving, more than ice cream
- **Blood Sugar Impact:** Severe spike despite "healthy" marketing
- **Better Alternative:** Unsweetened coconut yogurt or kefir

Cheese (Processed)

- **Types to Avoid:** American cheese, cheese spreads, processed cheese products
- **Why They're Harmful:** Artificial ingredients, preservatives, and inflammatory proteins
- **Blood Sugar Impact:** Minimal direct impact, but worsens insulin resistance
- **Better Alternative:** Raw, grass-fed cheese in small amounts

TIER 3: THE HIDDEN SABOTEURS

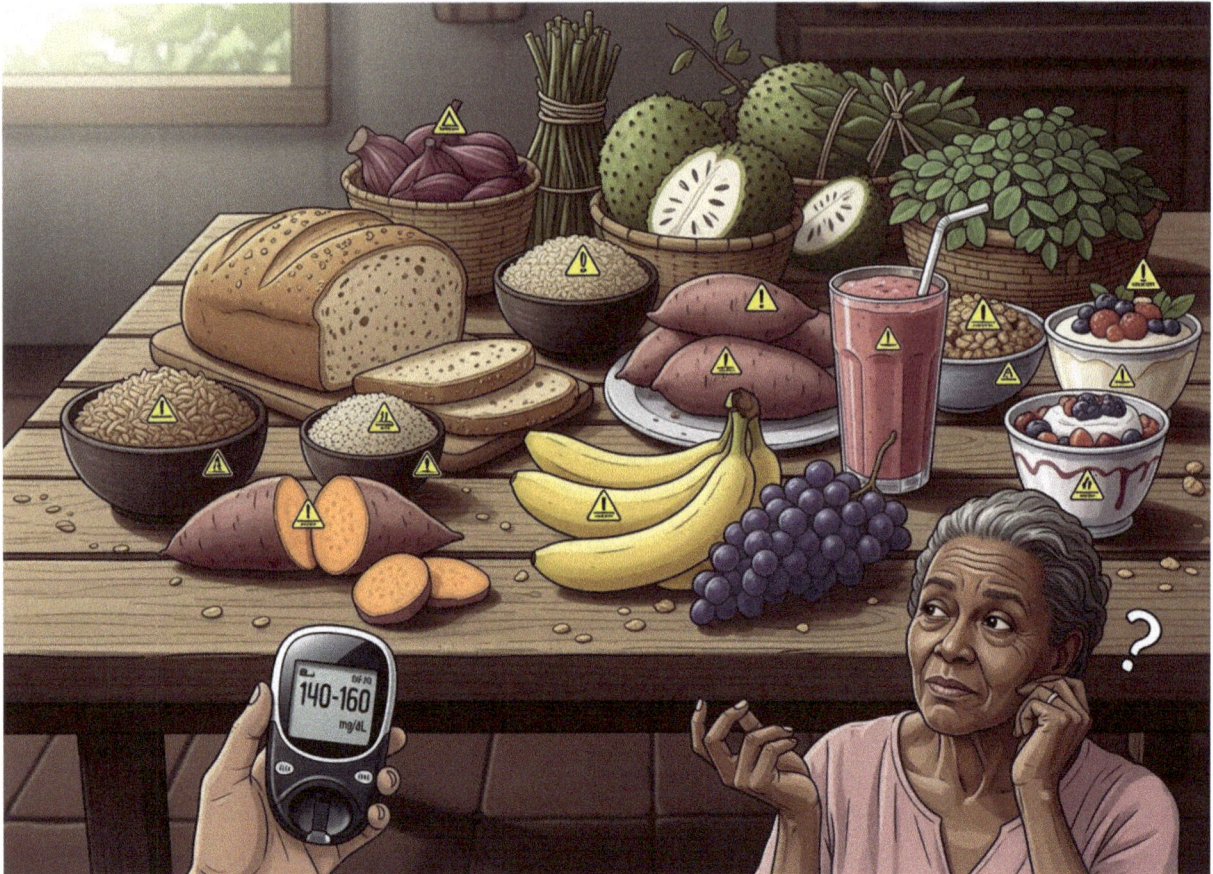

These foods are often considered "healthy" but can sabotage diabetes reversal efforts.

FRUITS (HIGH SUGAR)

Tropical Fruits

- **Types to Limit:** Pineapple, mango, papaya, banana, grapes
- **Why They're Problematic:** Very high in fructose, causing significant blood sugar spikes
- **Blood Sugar Impact:** 50-80 point spike, followed by a crash and cravings
- **The Natural Sugar Myth:** Natural doesn't mean safe for diabetics

Dried Fruits

- **Concentrated Sugar Bombs:** All water removed, sugar concentrated 5-10x
- **Types to Avoid:** Raisins, dates, dried cranberries, fruit leather
- **Blood Sugar Impact:** Severe and sustained elevation
- **Hidden Sources:** Trail mixes, granolas, "healthy" snack bars

Fruit Juices

- **Worse Than Soda:** Often higher in sugar than soft drinks
- **Types to Avoid:** All fruit juices, even "fresh" and "natural"
- **Blood Sugar Impact:** Rapid spike to 200+ mg/dL
- **The Fiber Fallacy:** Juicing removes beneficial fiber that slows absorption

LEGUMES AND BEANS

High-Starch Legumes

- **Types to Limit:** Kidney beans, black beans, pinto beans, chickpeas
- **Why They're Problematic:** High in starches that convert to glucose
- **Blood Sugar Impact:** Moderate but sustained elevation for 2-3 hours
- **Individual Variation:** Some diabetics tolerate small amounts, while others cannot

Soy Products

- **Types to Avoid:** Tofu, tempeh, soy milk, edamame
- **Why They're Harmful:** Phytoestrogens disrupt hormones, often GMO, high in lectins
- **Blood Sugar Impact:** Variable but often significant
- **Thyroid Disruption:** Can worsen hypothyroidism common in diabetics

THE BEVERAGE SABOTEURS

ALCOHOLIC BEVERAGES

Beer

- **The Liquid Bread:** Extremely high in carbohydrates
- **Blood Sugar Impact:** Severe spike followed by a dangerous low
- **Metabolic Damage:** Disrupts liver glucose regulation for 12-24 hours
- **No Safe Amount:** Even "light" beer causes problems

Sweet Wines and Cocktails

- **Hidden Sugar Bombs:** Often 20-40g sugar per drink
- **Blood Sugar Impact:** Unpredictable swings, dangerous lows hours later
- **Liver Stress:** Alcohol metabolism interferes with glucose regulation
- **Sleep Disruption:** Worsens sleep quality, affecting next-day blood sugar

CAFFEINATED BEVERAGES

Soft Drinks and Sodas

- **The Obvious Culprits:** 35-40g sugar per 12 oz serving

- **Blood Sugar Impact:** Rapid spike to 250+ mg/dL
- **Addiction Potential:** More addictive than many drugs
- **Diet Versions:** Artificial sweeteners worsen glucose tolerance

Energy Drinks

- **The Double Whammy:** High sugar plus caffeine crash
- **Blood Sugar Impact:** Extreme spike followed by severe crash
- **Adrenal Stress:** Worsens stress hormone imbalance
- **Heart Risks:** Dangerous for diabetics with cardiovascular issues

Fancy Coffee Drinks

- **Hidden Sugar Sources:** Flavored syrups, whipped cream, milk
- **Sugar Content:** Often 30-50g per large drink
- **Blood Sugar Impact:** Severe morning spike, disrupts entire day
- **Better Alternative:** Black coffee with coconut oil or MCT oil

THE RESTAURANT AND TAKEOUT TRAPS

FAST FOOD DISASTERS

Burgers and Sandwiches

- **The Bun Problem:** Refined flour buns cause severe blood sugar spikes
- **Hidden Sugars:** Condiments, pickles, processed meats
- **Inflammatory Oils:** Cooked in toxic vegetable oils
- **Portion Distortion:** Massive servings overwhelm metabolism

Pizza

- **The Perfect Storm:** Refined flour crust, sugary sauce, processed cheese
- **Blood Sugar Impact:** Sustained elevation for 4-6 hours
- **Inflammatory Response:** Multiple inflammatory ingredients combined
- **No Healthy Versions:** Even "cauliflower crust" versions are often problematic

Chinese Takeout

- **Sugar-Coated Everything:** Most sauces are loaded with sugar and corn starch
- **Hidden Carbs:** Breading, thickeners, rice, noodles
- **MSG Problems:** Can trigger insulin resistance in sensitive individuals
- **Vegetable Oil Overload:** Everything cooked in inflammatory oils

THE TIMING TRAP

LATE-NIGHT EATING

Why Timing Matters:

- Insulin sensitivity drops 50% after 8 PM
- Late eating disrupts circadian rhythms
- Interferes with growth hormone release
- Causes morning blood sugar spikes

Foods That Are Worse at Night:

- Any carbohydrates become more problematic
- Alcohol effects are magnified
- Even "healthy" foods can cause issues
- Snacking disrupts overnight fasting benefits

THE PORTION DECEPTION

Why "Just a Little" Doesn't Work:

The Metabolic Memory Effect:

- Small amounts of harmful foods trigger cravings for more
- Insulin resistance worsens with each exposure
- The inflammatory cascade lasts for hours
- Undoes progress from healing foods

The All-or-Nothing Principle:

- Complete elimination is easier than moderation
- Cravings disappear after 2-3 weeks of avoidance
- Taste preferences change toward healing foods
- Metabolic healing accelerates with complete avoidance

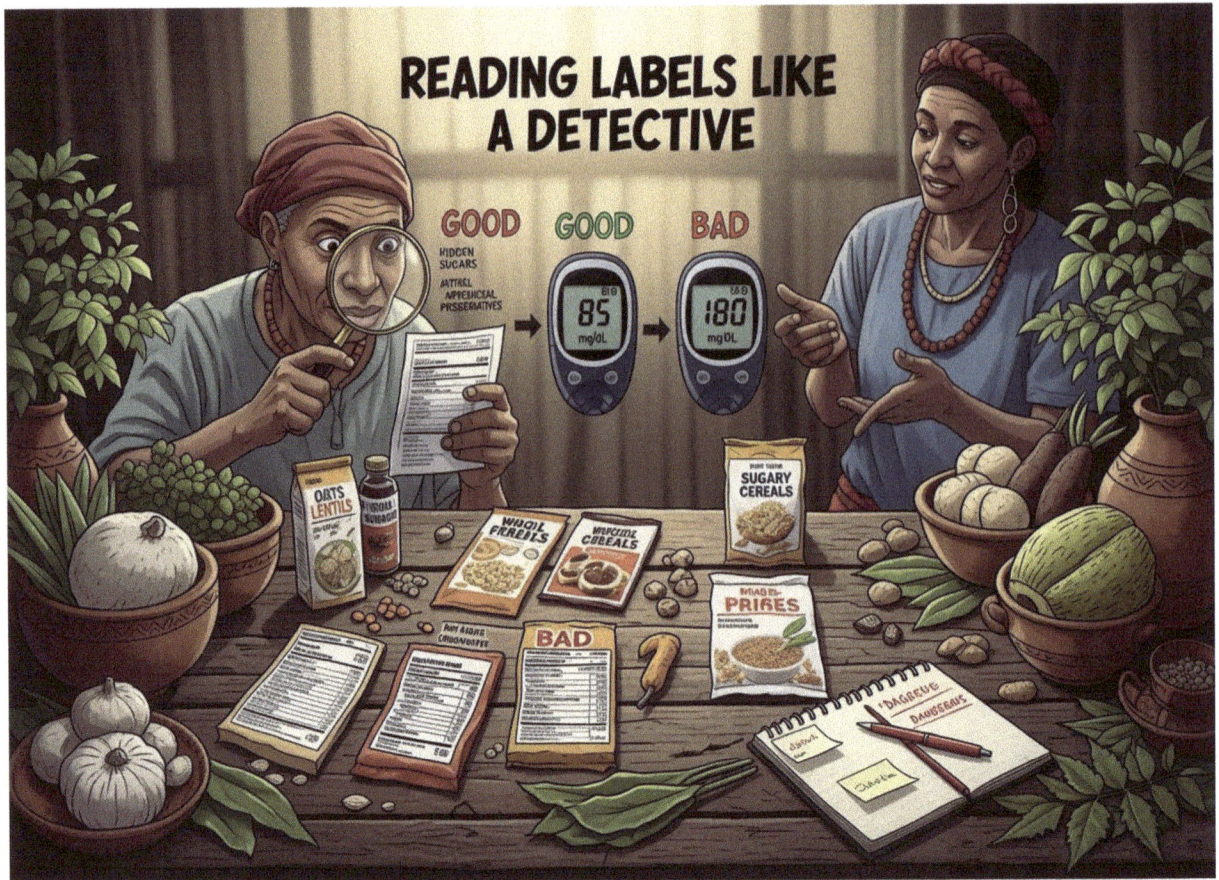

Hidden Sugar Names:

- Dextrose, maltose, sucrose, fructose
- Corn syrup, rice syrup, malt syrup
- Fruit juice concentrate, evaporated cane juice
- Barley malt, brown rice syrup
- Anything ending in "-ose"

Inflammatory Oil Code Words:

- "Vegetable oil" (usually soybean)
- "Natural flavors" (often contain oils)
- "Partially hydrogenated" (trans fats)
- "Interesterified fats" (new trans fat alternative)

Starch and Flour Disguises:

- "Wheat flour" (refined white flour)
- "Enriched flour" (stripped and artificially fortified)
- "Multigrain" (often mostly refined flour)
- "Modified food starch" (blood sugar spiker)

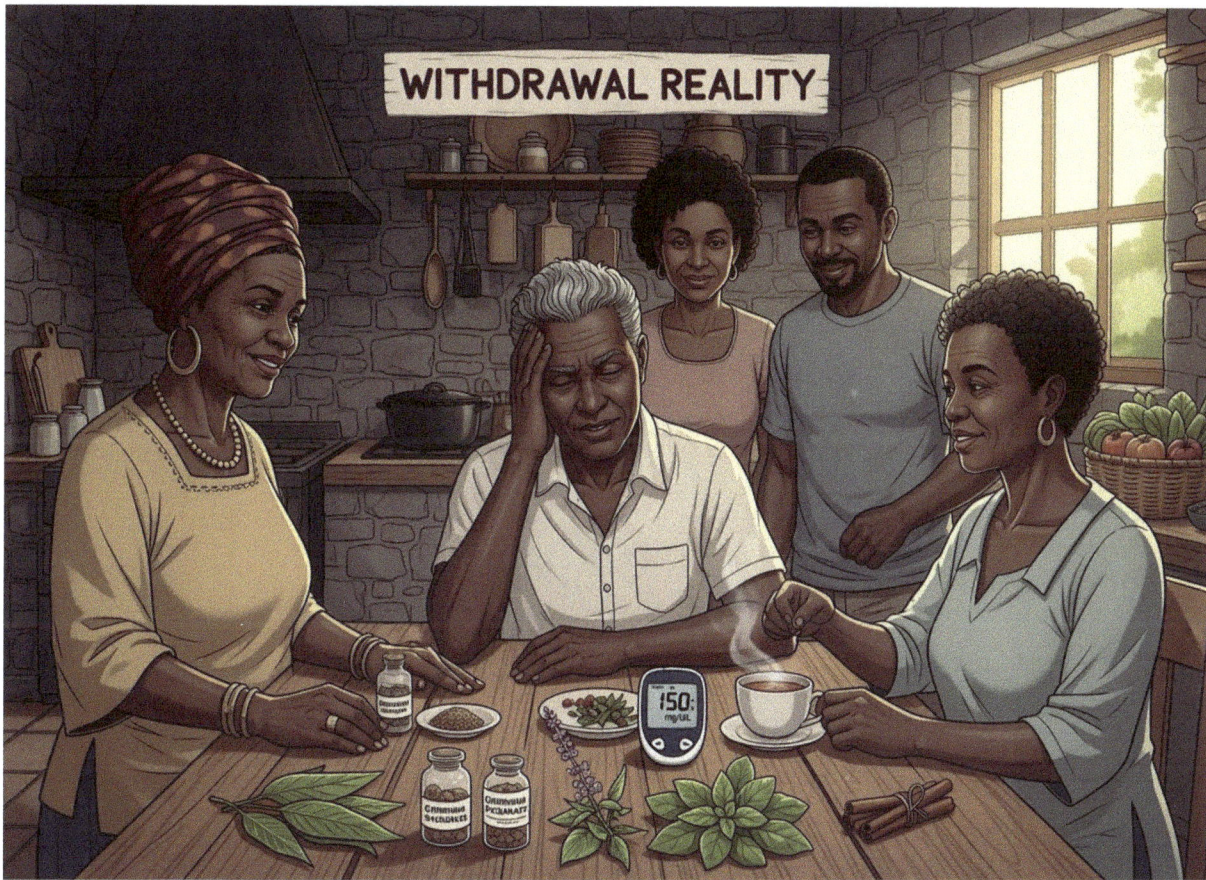

What to Expect When Eliminating Harmful Foods:

Week 1-2: The Detox Phase

- Intense cravings for eliminated foods
- Possible headaches and fatigue
- Mood swings and irritability
- Sleep disruptions

Week 3-4: The Turning Point

- Cravings begin to diminish
- Energy levels start improving
- Blood sugar becomes more stable
- Taste preferences begin changing

Month 2-3: The New Normal

- Former favorite foods lose appeal
- Natural hunger and satiety return
- Stable energy throughout the day
- Significant blood sugar improvements

SOCIAL PRESSURE AND FOOD PUSHERS

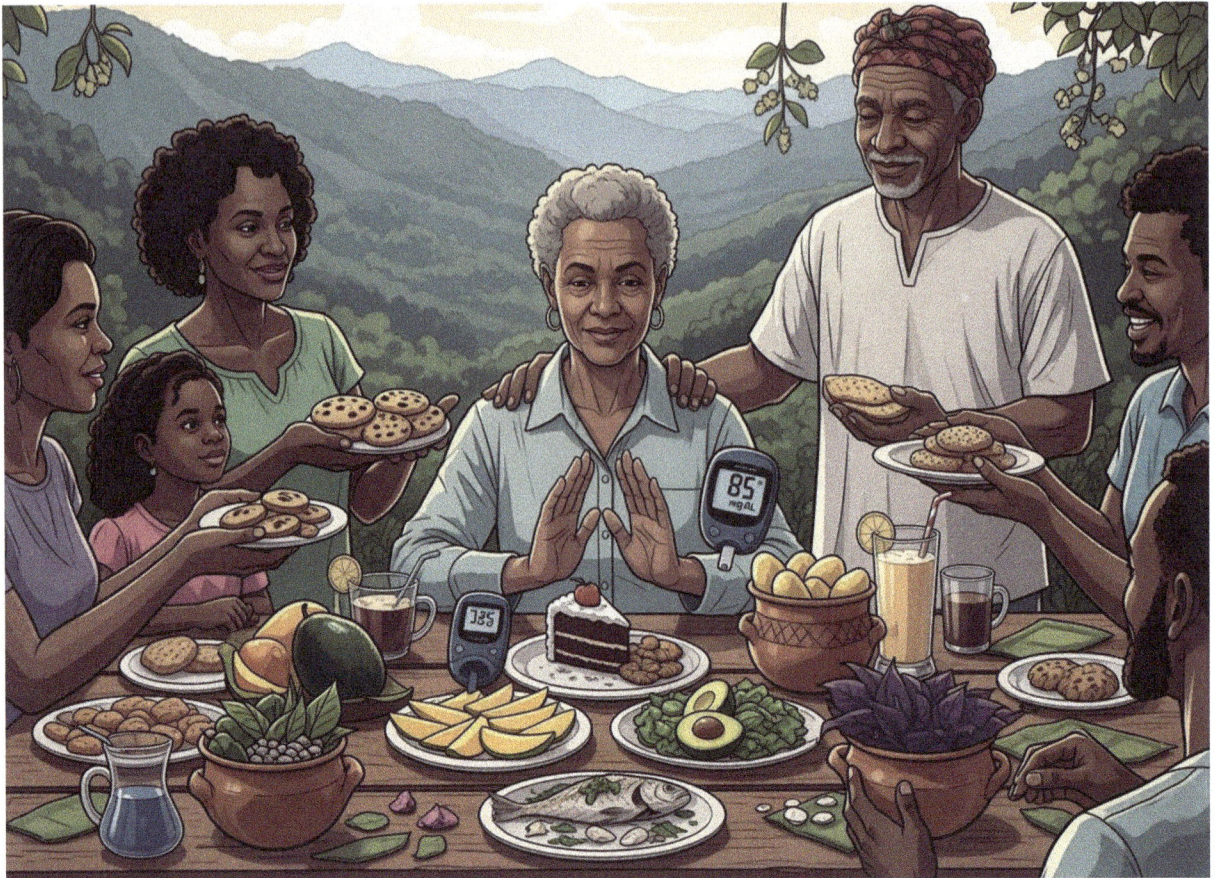

Handling Well-Meaning Saboteurs:

Family Gatherings:

- "I'm following a specific health protocol."
- "My doctor has me on a special diet."
- "I feel so much better eating this way."
- Bring your own healing foods to share

Work Situations:

- "I'm managing a health condition."
- "Sugar makes me feel terrible."
- "I prefer to eat this way."
- Keep healing snacks at your desk

Friend Pressure:

- "I'm committed to reversing my diabetes."
- "This is working so well for m.e"

- "I don't want to undo my progress."
- Suggest activities that don't center around food

EMERGENCY STRATEGIES

When You're Tempted:

The 10-Minute Rule:

- Wait 10 minutes before eating the harmful food
- Drink 16 oz of water with lemon
- Take 5 deep breaths
- Remind yourself of your why

The Substitution Strategy:

- Have healing alternatives ready
- Raw nuts instead of chips
- Herbal tea instead of soda
- Avocado instead of bread

The Consequence Visualization:

- Picture your blood sugar spiking
- Remember how you felt on medications
- Visualize your health goals
- Think about people counting on you

REAL SUCCESS STORIES

Maria's Elimination Victory: "The hardest part was giving up bread. I thought I couldn't live without it. But after three weeks, I stopped craving it completely. Now, when I smell fresh bread, it doesn't even appeal to me. My blood sugars dropped 80 points just from eliminating the foods that were sabotaging me."

John's Restaurant Strategy: "I used to think I couldn't eat out anymore. Then I learned to order strategically - grilled fish with vegetables, salads with olive oil, and steak with no sides. Most restaurants can accommodate you if you're clear about your needs. My friends barely notice I'm eating differently."

YOUR ELIMINATION STRATEGY

The 30-Day Complete Elimination:

- Remove all Tier 1 foods immediately
- Eliminate Tier 2 foods by day 7

- Address Tier 3 foods by day 14
- Focus on healing foods only

Tracking Your Progress:

- Daily blood sugar readings
- Energy levels and mood
- Cravings intensity (1-10 scale)
- Sleep quality improvements
- Weight and body composition changes

THE LIBERATION MINDSET

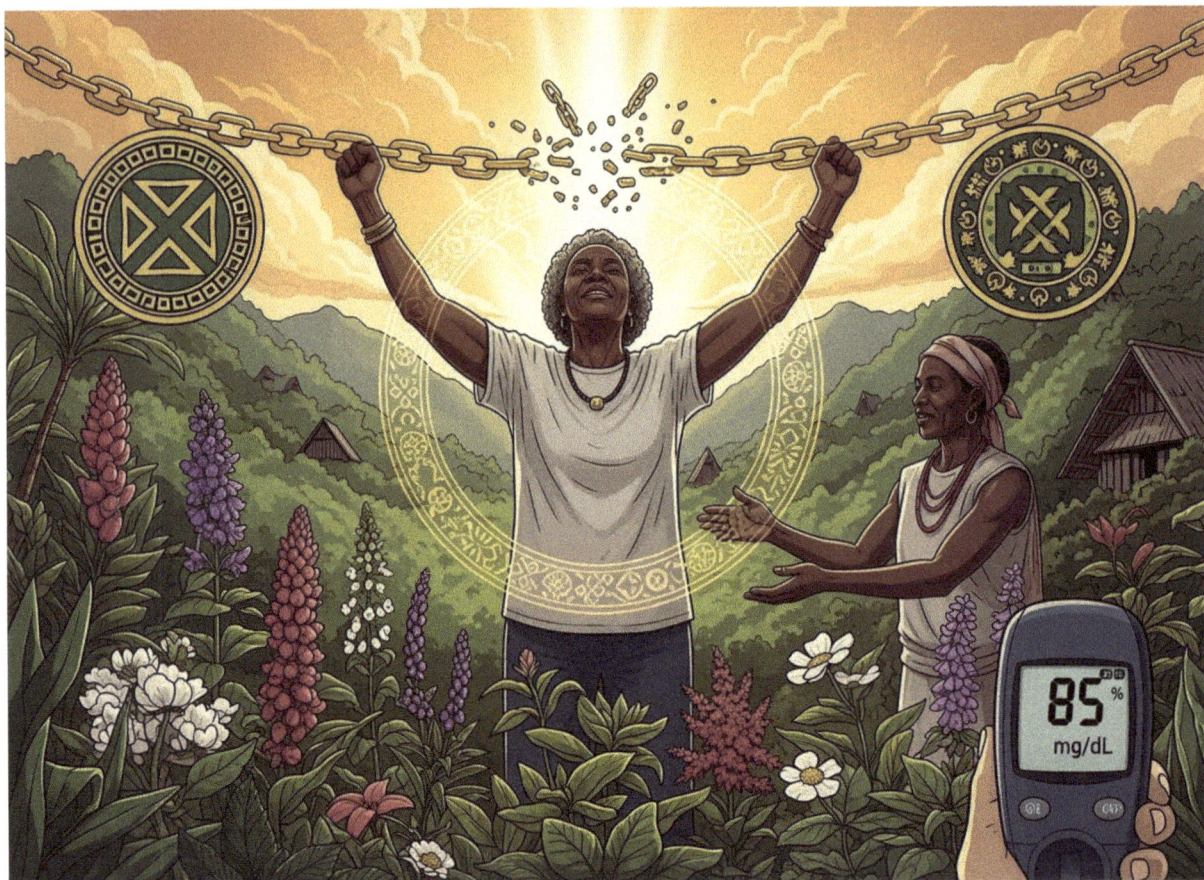

Reframing Food Elimination:

Instead of thinking "I can't have that," think:

- "I choose not to poison myself."

- "I'm free from food addiction."
- "I nourish my body with healing foods"
- "I'm reversing my diabetes naturally."

This isn't deprivation - it's liberation from the foods that created your diabetes and kept you trapped in medication dependence.

YOUR PERSONALIZED ELIMINATION PLAN

Individual challenges may include:

- Cultural food traditions
- Family cooking and eating patterns
- Work and travel food situations
- Budget and accessibility constraints

Schedule Your FREE 15-Minute Consultation

During this call, we'll create a personalized elimination strategy that addresses your specific challenges and ensures the successful removal of all diabetes-sabotaging foods.

THE COMMITMENT TO ELIMINATION

Eliminating harmful foods is more than just a dietary change - it's a declaration of independence from the foods that contributed to your diabetes and a commitment to the healing foods that will help reverse it.

Every harmful food you refuse is a victory. Every healing food you choose is a step forward. Every day you maintain this commitment is a step closer to complete diabetes reversal.

In the next chapter, we'll explore your complete 4-month transformation timeline - the week-by-week roadmap to diabetes freedom.

CHAPTER 12
YOUR 4-MONTH
TRANSFORMATION TIMELINE

"The journey from diabetes to freedom follows a predictable path. Understanding what to expect each week gives you the confidence to stay committed when challenges arise."

After helping over 10,000 people reverse their diabetes using the Sweet Blood Protocol, I can tell you exactly what to expect during your 16-week transformation journey.

Every person's body responds differently, but the patterns are remarkably consistent. Understanding these patterns will give you the confidence to trust the process, especially during the challenging early weeks when your body is adjusting to the healing process.

This timeline is based on real client experiences and 65+ years of clinical observation. Your individual results may vary, but 80% of people following the protocol experience similar progression patterns.

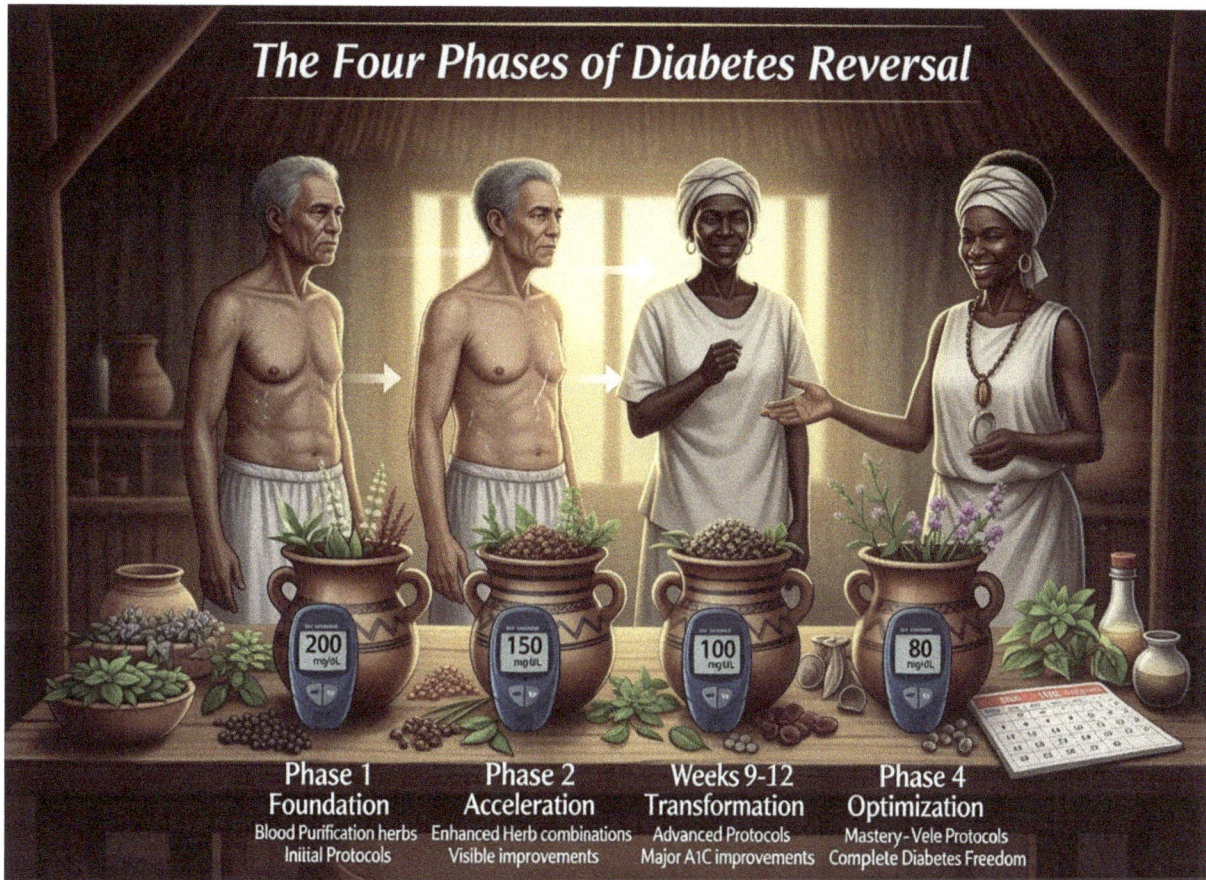

The Four Phases of Diabetes Reversal

Phase 1 Foundation	Phase 2 Acceleration	Weeks 9-12 Transformation	Phase 4 Optimization
Blood Purification herbs Initial Protocols	Enhanced Herb combinations Visible improvements	Advanced Protocols Major A1C improvements	Mastery-Vele Protocols Complete Diabetes Freedom

Phase 1: Foundation (Weeks 1-4)

- Initial detoxification and metabolic adjustment
- Blood sugar begins stabilizing
- Energy levels start improving
- Medication adjustments may begin

Phase 2: Acceleration (Weeks 5-8)

- Dramatic blood sugar improvements
- Significant medication reductions
- Visible physical changes
- Increased confidence and motivation

Phase 3: Transformation (Weeks 9-12)

- Major metabolic shifts
- Most medications eliminated
- Complete energy restoration
- Physical transformation visible to others

Phase 4: Mastery (Weeks 13-16)

- Blood sugar normalization
- Medication freedom achieved
- A1C in normal range
- Complete diabetes reversal documented

WEEK 1: THE FOUNDATION BEGINS

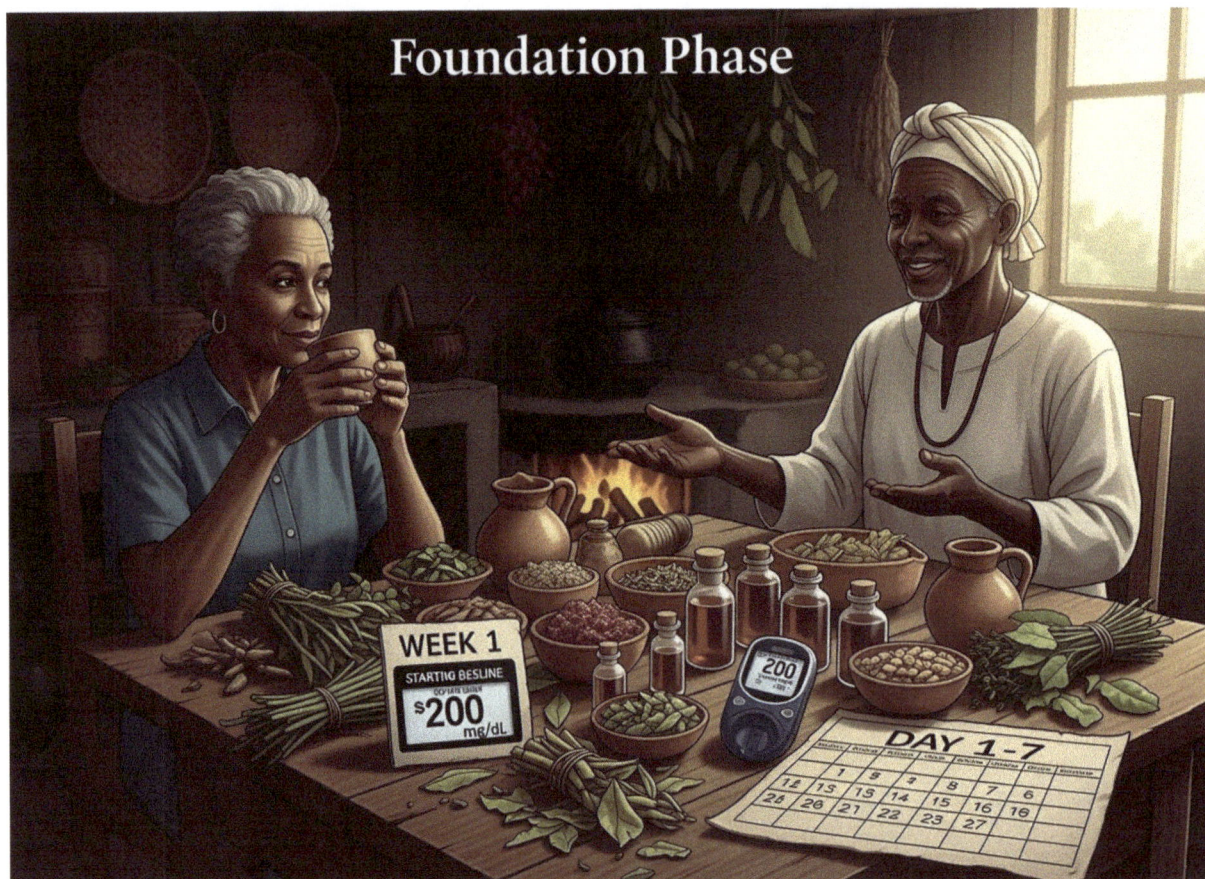

What You're Starting:

- Morning ritual with blood purification tea
- Pre-meal supplements (gymnema, berberine, digestive enzymes)
- Elimination of all harmful foods
- Gentle post-meal movement
- Blood sugar monitoring 4x daily

What to Expect:

Days 1-3: The Initial Shock. Your body is adjusting to the absence of sugar and processed foods. This is normal and temporary.

- Blood sugar readings may be erratic
- Possible headaches from sugar withdrawal
- Increased urination as toxins are released
- Some fatigue as your metabolism shifts
- Strong cravings for familiar foods

Days 4-7: Early Signs of Hope

- Morning blood sugar begins dropping (typically 10-20 points)
- Post-meal spikes start reducing
- Sleep quality may begin improving
- Energy levels become more stable
- Cravings start diminishing

Milestone Markers:

- First normal blood sugar reading (even if brief)
- Sleeping through the night without bathroom trips
- Waking up with more energy than usual
- Clothes feel slightly looser

Common Challenges:

- Intense sugar cravings (especially days 3-5)
- Family resistance to dietary changes
- Doubt about whether "natural" approaches work
- Impatience with the pace of change

Victory Celebrations:

- Every 10-point drop in morning blood sugar
- Each day is completed without harmful foods
- First compliment about looking healthier
- First medication adjustment discussion with the doctor

Success Story - Week 1: *"I was skeptical that herbs could help my 15-year diabetes, but by day 6, my morning readings dropped from 240 to 195. That 45-point improvement in less than a week gave me the hope I needed to continue."* - Margaret, Age 58

WEEK 2: BUILDING MOMENTUM

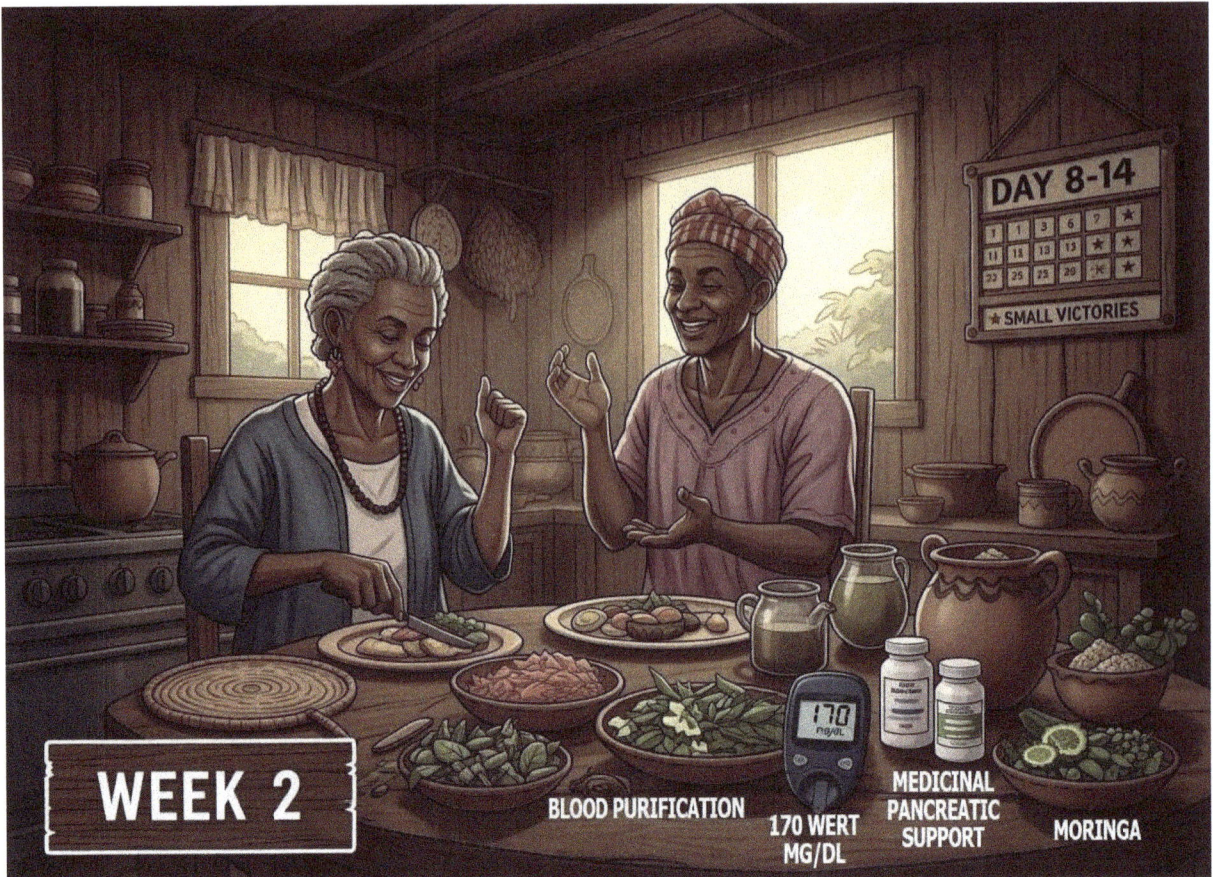

What You're Adding:

- Evening restoration protocol
- Extended post-meal walks (15-20 minutes)
- Stress management techniques
- More variety in healing foods

What to Expect:

Physical Changes:

- Continued blood sugar improvements (20-40 points from baseline)
- Reduced sugar cravings (50% less intense)
- Better digestion and elimination
- Improved circulation in hands and feet
- Natural weight loss begins (2-4 pounds)

Mental/Emotional Changes:

- Increased confidence in the protocol
- Better mood stability throughout the day
- Reduced anxiety about blood sugar readings
- Growing excitement about progress
- Hope replacing fear

Milestone Markers:

- First post-meal reading under 180 mg/dL
- Sleeping 6+ hours without interruption
- Walking up stairs without breathlessness
- Noticing improved skin tone

Common Challenges:

- Social eating situations become difficult
- Others are questioning your "extreme" approach
- Plateau in blood sugar improvements
- Impatience with gradual progress

Victory Celebrations:

- First week completed successfully
- Clothes fitting better
- Compliments from family/friends
- Doctors' surprise at improvements

WEEK 3: THE TURNING POINT

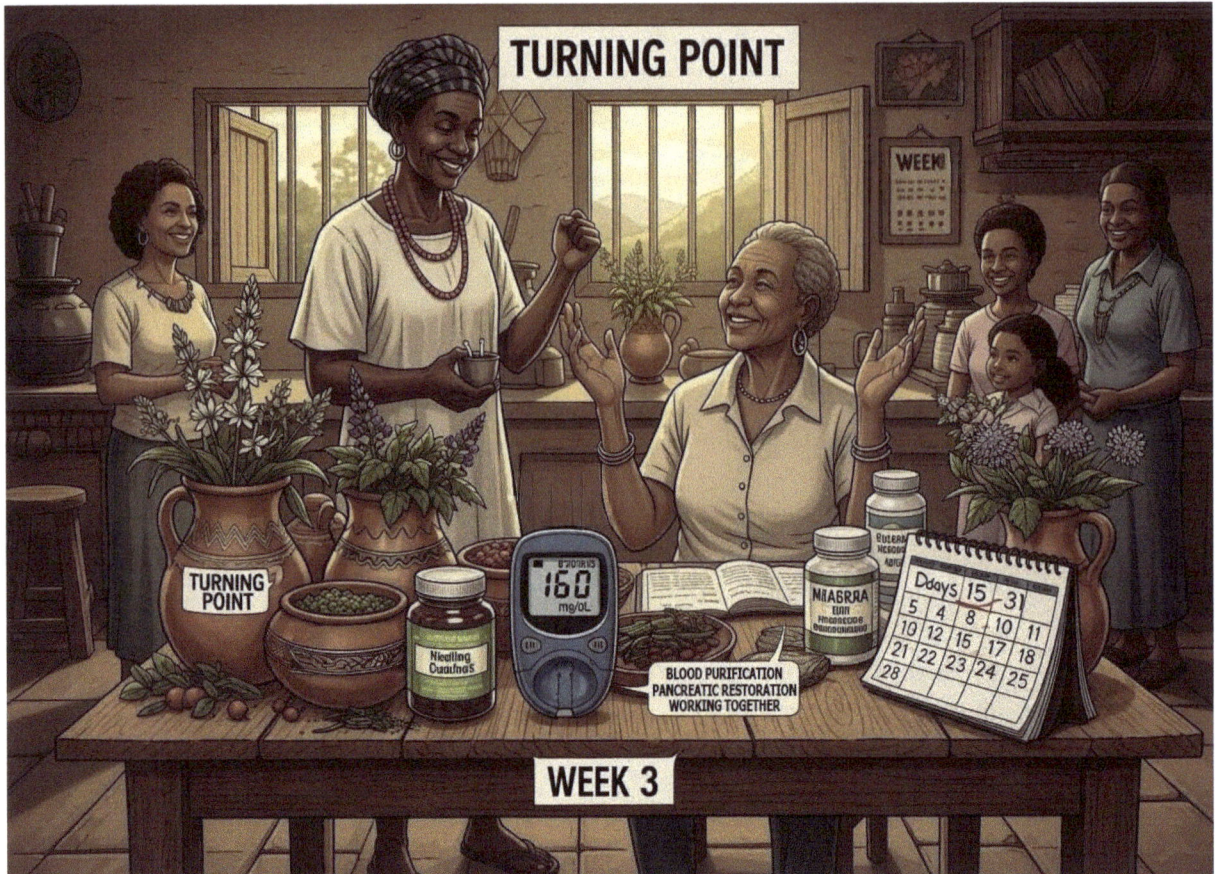

What's Happening: This is often the breakthrough week when people realize the protocol is truly working.

What to Expect:

Breakthrough Moments:

- First completely normal blood sugar reading in months/years
- Waking up refreshed instead of exhausted
- Realizing you forgot to think about food for hours
- Feeling genuinely hopeful about your health future

Physical Improvements:

- Morning readings consistently under 150 mg/dL
- Post-meal spikes rarely exceed 160 mg/dL
- Natural weight loss becomes noticeable (4-7 pounds total)
- Better wound healing and reduced infections
- Improved vision clarity

Energy Transformation:

- Sustained energy throughout the day
- No more afternoon crashes
- Ability to be active after meals
- Mental clarity and focus are returning

Milestone Markers:

- First A1C projection showing significant improvement
- Doctor discussing medication reduction
- Others commenting on your transformation
- Feeling genuinely excited about your health

Medication Alert: Many people need their first medication adjustment during week 3. Work closely with your healthcare provider to reduce medications safely as blood sugars improve.

Success Story - Week 3: *"On day 18, I woke up with a blood sugar of 98 - the first time in 5 years it was under 100. I actually cried tears of joy. That's when I knew this protocol was really working."* - David, Age 52

WEEK 4: ESTABLISHING THE NEW NORMAL

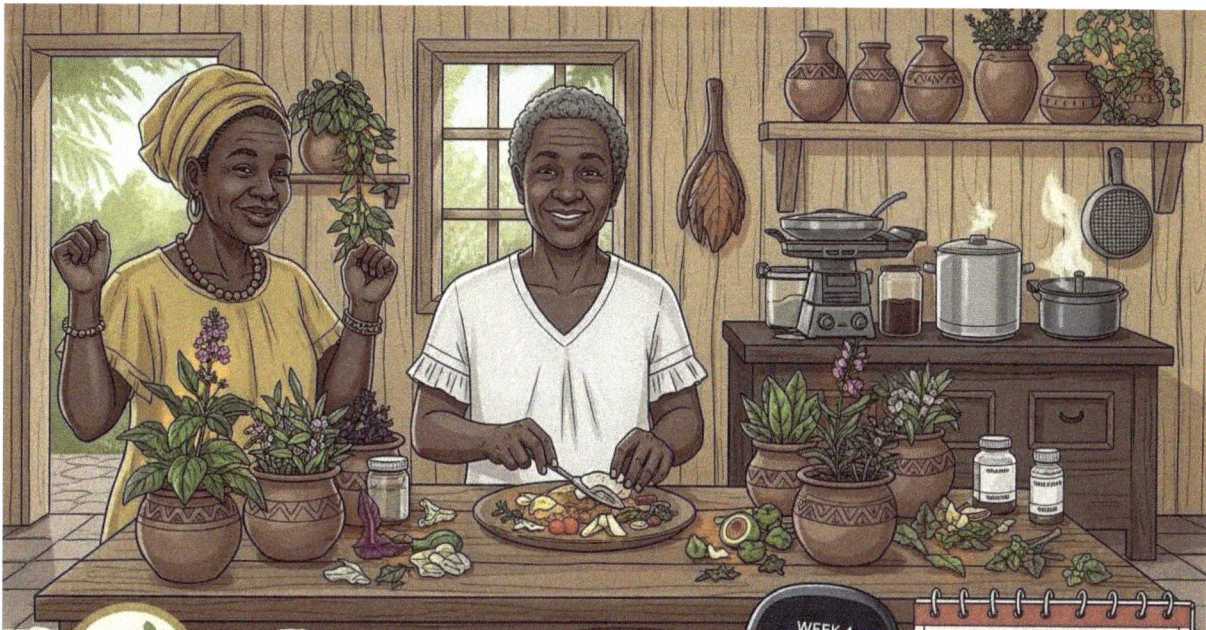

What You're Mastering:

- Consistent daily routines are becoming automatic
- Healthy food choices feel natural
- Stress management is becoming habitual
- Confidence in your healing ability is growing

What to Expect:

Metabolic Stabilization:

- More predictable blood sugar patterns
- Reduced variability in daily readings
- Stable energy from morning to night
- Improved insulin sensitivity markers

Lifestyle Integration:

- Protocols feel less like "work" and more like routine
- Family begins adapting to new eating patterns
- Social situations become more manageable
- Increased motivation to continue

Physical Changes:

- Consistent weight loss (6-10 pounds total)
- Improved muscle tone and strength
- Better skin, hair, and nail health
- Reduced inflammation throughout the body

Milestone Markers:

- One full month of protocol completion
- Significant medication reduction achieved
- A1C projection showing 0.5-1.0 point improvement
- Others are asking about your "secret"

Month 1 Assessment:

- Schedule comprehensive lab work
- Review progress with the healthcare provider
- Document transformation with photos
- Plan for Phase 2 acceleration

WEEKS 5-6:

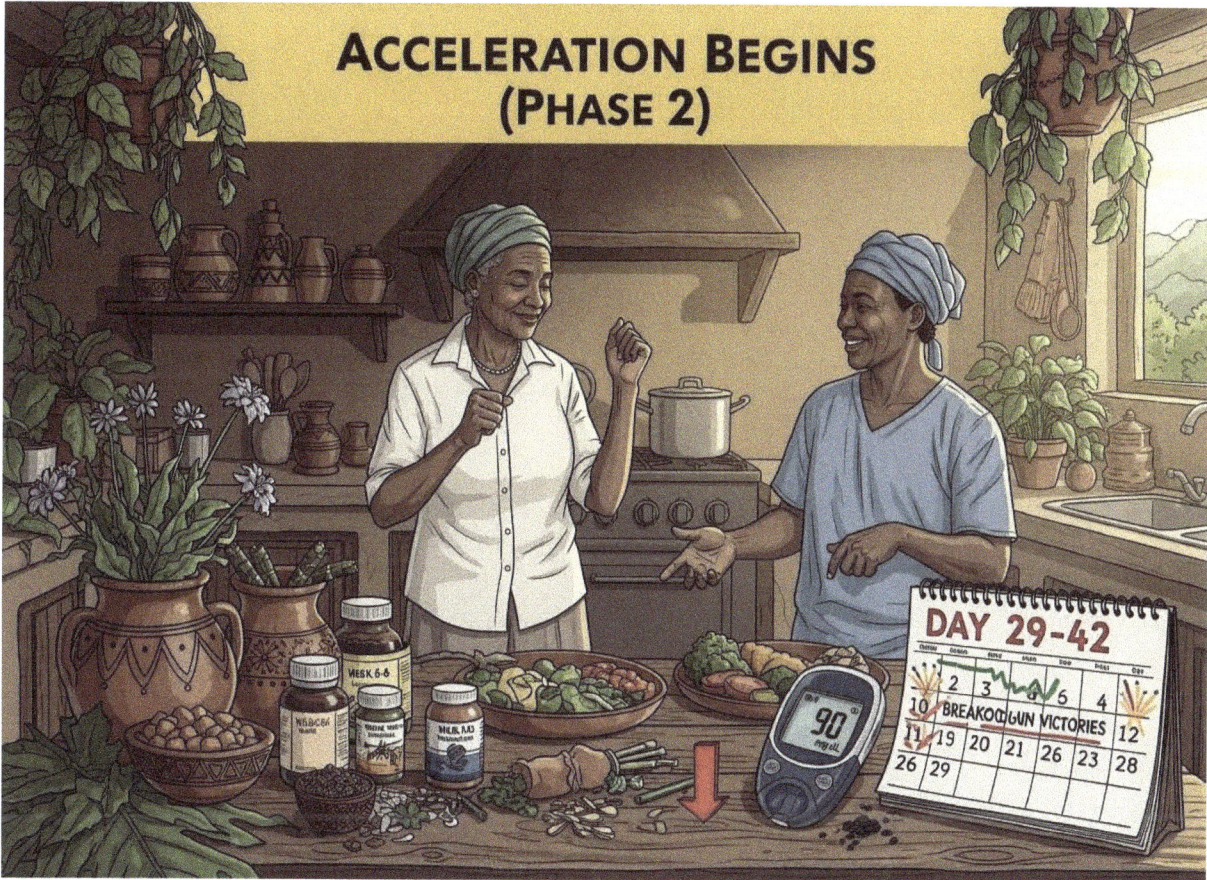

What's Different: You're entering the acceleration phase, where changes happen more rapidly and dramatically.

What to Expect:

Dramatic Improvements:

- Consistent normal morning readings (80-120 mg/dL)
- Post-meal spikes become minimal (under 140 mg/dL)
- Natural weight loss accelerates
- Energy levels are fully restored to youthful levels

Physical Transformation:

- Significant visible weight loss (8-15 pounds total)
- Better skin tone and clarity
- Improved muscle definition
- Enhanced mental clarity and memory

Medical Milestones:

- First major medication elimination
- Doctor's amazement at your progress
- Lab work showing dramatic improvements
- Blood pressure normalization

Milestone Markers:

- First completely medication-free day
- Running or exercising without breathlessness
- Fitting into clothes from years ago
- Others are asking if you've had surgery

Success Story - Weeks 5-6: *"My doctor couldn't believe my 6-week lab results. My A1C dropped from 9.2 to 7.1, and I was off two of my four medications. He said he'd never seen an improvement that dramatic without increasing medications - I was eliminating them!"* - Patricia, Age 61

WEEKS 7-8: TRANSFORMATION VISIBLE

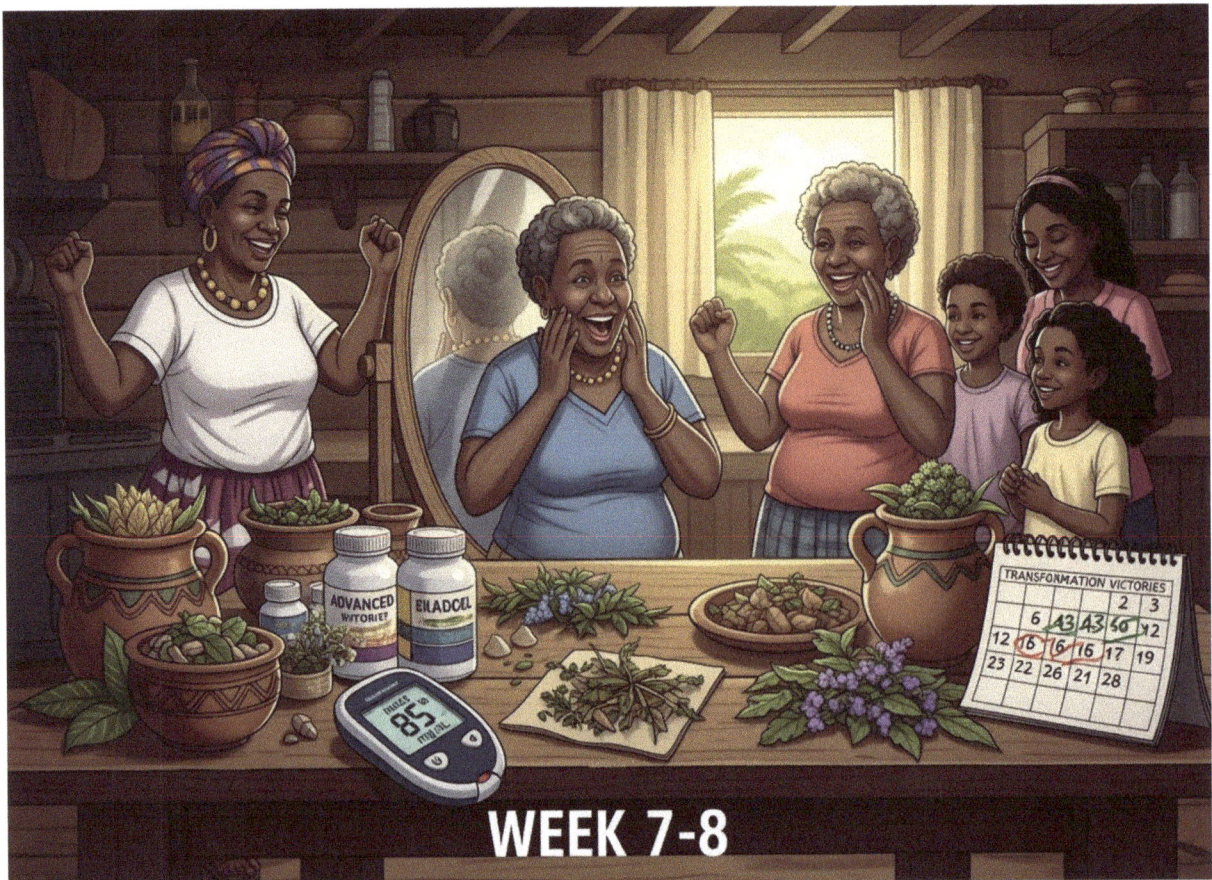

WEEK 7-8

What Others Notice:

- Significant weight loss and improved appearance
- Increased energy and vitality
- Better mood and positive outlook
- Obvious reduction in medications

What You're Experiencing:

- Stable blood sugar without constant effort
- Natural appetite regulation
- Improved sleep quality and dream recall
- Increased physical activity tolerance

Physical Changes:

- Major weight loss visible (12-20 pounds total)
- Improved cardiovascular fitness
- Better flexibility and mobility
- Reduced pain and inflammation

Milestone Markers:

- Two months of successful protocol completion
- Multiple medications eliminated
- A1C projection under 7.0
- Planning activities you couldn't do before

The 8-Week Celebration: This is a major milestone worth celebrating. You've proven to yourself and others that diabetes reversal is possible.

WEEKS 9-10: ENTERING TRANSFORMATION PHASE (PHASE 3)

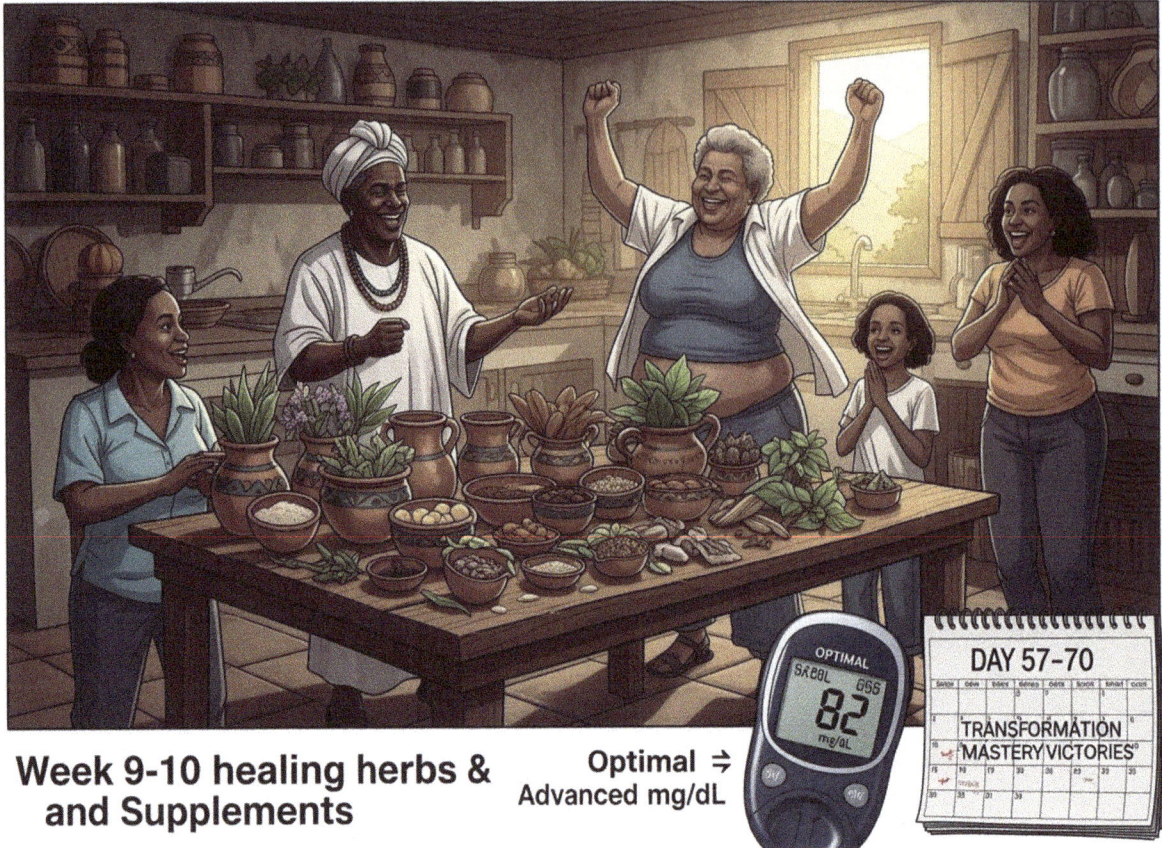

Week 9-10 healing herbs & and Supplements

Optimal ⇒ Advanced mg/dL

OPTIMAL

82 mg/dL

DAY 57-70

TRANSFORMATION MASTERY VICTORIES

What's Different: You're entering the transformation phase, where your body completes its metabolic healing.

Physical Transformation:

- Major weight loss is clearly visible (15-25 pounds total)
- Improved body composition (less fat, more muscle)
- Better cardiovascular health markers
- Enhanced immune function

Metabolic Transformation:

- Insulin sensitivity dramatically improved
- Pancreatic function was significantly restored
- Liver function optimized
- Inflammation markers normalized

Lifestyle Changes:

- Exercise becomes enjoyable rather than difficult
- Healthy eating feels completely natural
- Energy levels rival those of decades ago
- Confidence in your health is unshakeable

Milestone Markers:

- A1C projection approaching normal range
- Most diabetes medications have been eliminated
- Others are asking about your transformation
- Planning future health goals

WEEKS 11-12: MAJOR MILESTONES

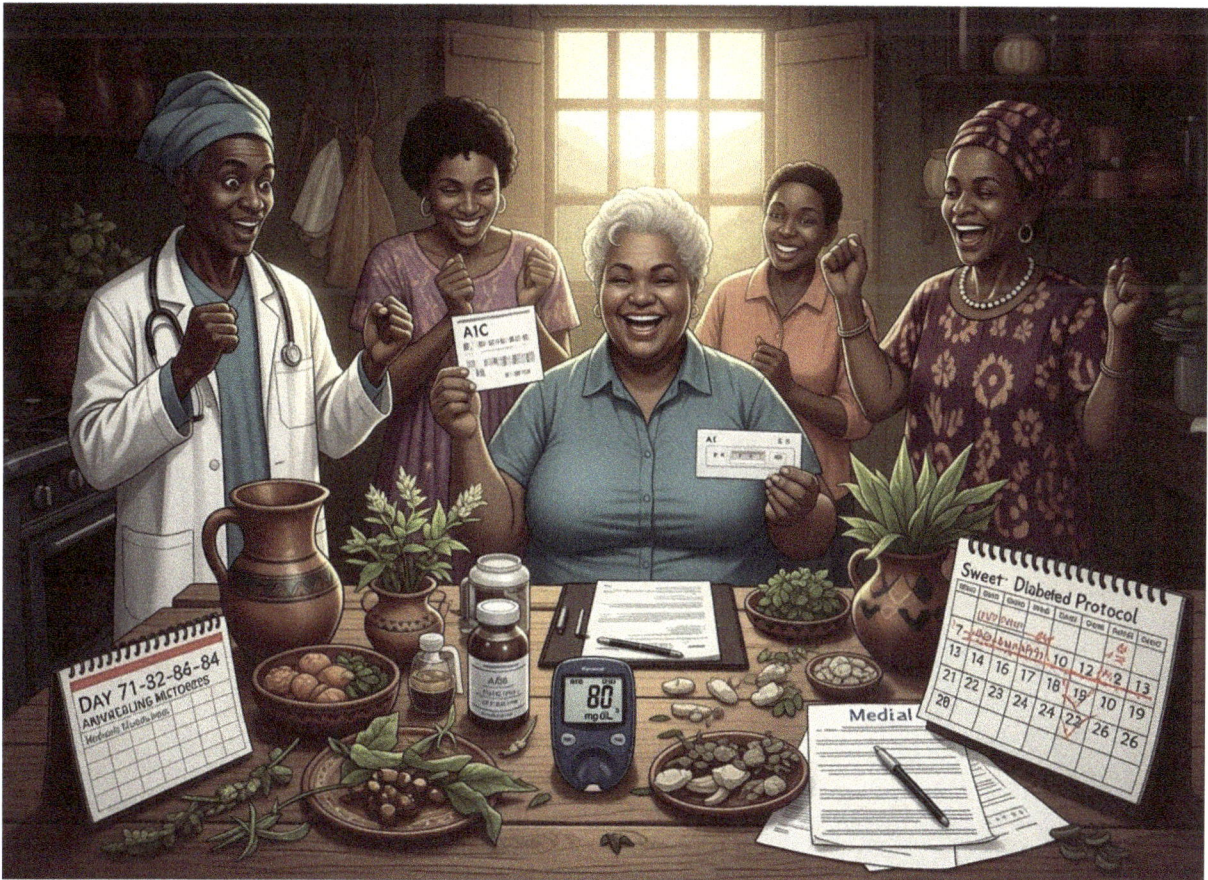

What You're Achieving:

- Near-normal blood sugar patterns consistently
- Minimal or no diabetes medications needed
- Complete energy restoration
- Confidence in long-term success

Health Improvements Beyond Diabetes:

- Blood pressure normalization
- Cholesterol profile improvements
- Better kidney function markers
- Improved nerve function and sensation

Physical Achievements:

- Significant weight loss (20-30 pounds total)
- Improved physical fitness and endurance
- Better balance and coordination
- Youthful energy and vitality

Milestone Markers:

- Three months of transformation have been completed
- A1C projection in normal range
- 75-90% medication reduction achieved
- Planning a celebration of your success

3-Month Lab Results: Most people see dramatic improvements in their 3-month lab work:

- A1C drops of 2-4 points
- Improved lipid profiles
- Better kidney function markers
- Reduced inflammation indicators

WEEKS 13-14: OPTIMIZATION PHASE (PHASE 4)

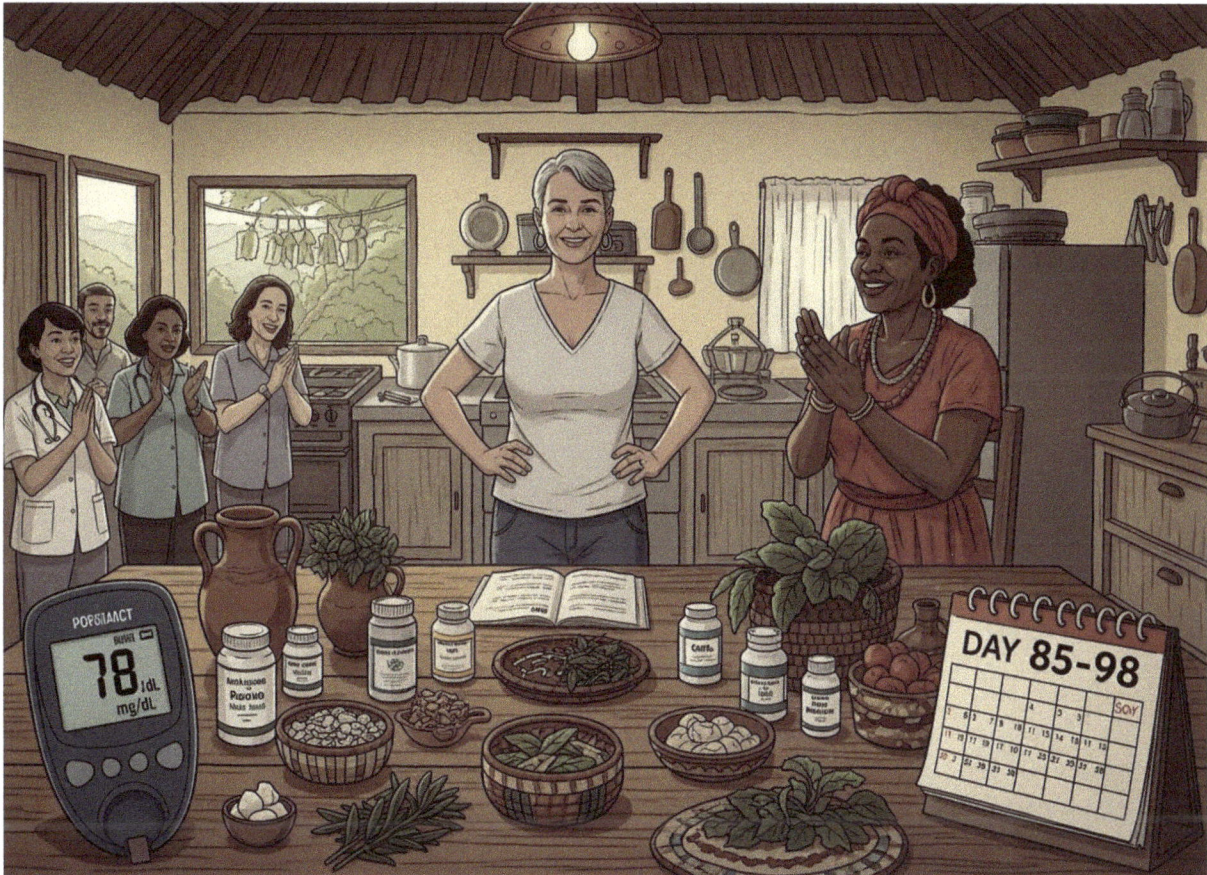

What's Happening: You're entering the final phase where your body optimizes its new healthy state.

Metabolic Optimization:

- Blood sugar patterns completely normalized
- Insulin sensitivity is fully restored
- Pancreatic function optimized
- Complete metabolic transformation achieved

Physical Optimization:

- Weight stabilized at a healthy level (25-35 pounds lost total)
- Muscle tone and strength optimized
- Cardiovascular fitness at peak
- All body systems are functioning optimally

Milestone Markers:

- Preparing for final A1C testing
- Planning a medication-free future
- Others are inspired by your transformation
- Confidence in permanent success

WEEKS 15-16: DIABETES REVERSAL ACHIEVED

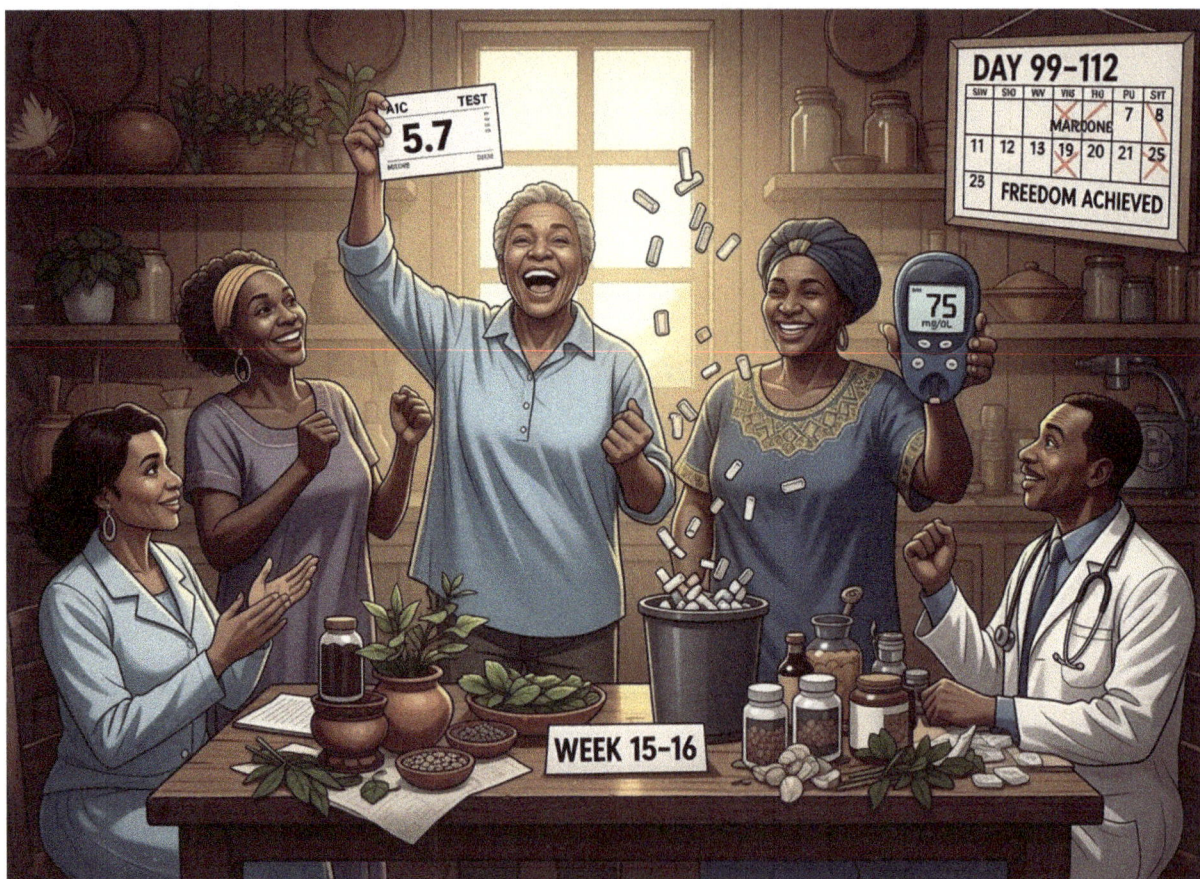

The Final Milestone:

- 4-month A1C testing confirms reversal
- Complete or near-complete medication freedom
- Full energy and vitality restoration
- Diabetes reversal officially documented

What to Expect:

- A1C below 5.7 (normal range)
- Minimal or no diabetes medications needed
- Stable weight at a healthy level
- Complete confidence in your health

The Victory Celebration:

- A1C in normal range (under 5.7)
- Medication freedom achieved (90-100% reduction)
- Total weight loss (25-40 pounds)
- Complete diabetes reversal documented

Success Story - Week 16: *"My 4-month A1C was 5.4 - completely normal! I went from taking 4 diabetes medications to taking none. My doctor said I no longer meet the criteria for diabetes. After 8 years of being diabetic, I'm finally free!"* - Robert, Age 49

TRACKING YOUR TRANSFORMATION

Daily Measurements:

- Fasting blood glucose (upon waking)
- Pre-meal readings (before the largest meal)
- Post-meal readings (2 hours after meals)
- Bedtime glucose levels
- Energy level (1-10 scale)
- Sleep quality assessment
- Overall well-being score

Weekly Assessments:

- Weight and body measurements
- Medication needs and changes
- Protocol compliance percentage
- Challenge identification and solutions
- Victory celebrations and milestones

Monthly Evaluations:

- Comprehensive lab work review
- Healthcare provider consultations
- Protocol adjustments and optimizations
- Progress photos and documentation
- Goal setting for next month

OVERCOMING COMMON PLATEAUS

Week 3-4 Plateau:

- **What's Happening:** Body adjusting to new metabolism
- **Normal Duration:** Usually resolves by week 5
- **What to Do:** Increase post-meal movement, stay consistent
- **Why It Happens:** Metabolic adaptation period

Week 7-8 Plateau:

- **What's Happening:** Need for protocol intensification
- **Normal Duration:** Breakthrough typically occurs week 9
- **What to Do:** Add weekly intensive protocols, optimize sleep
- **Why It Happens:** Body preparing for major transformation

Week 11-12 Plateau:

- **What's Happening:** Fine-tuning for final optimization
- **Normal Duration:** Final push leads to complete reversal
- **What to Do:** Focus on stress management, trust the process
- **Why It Happens:** Body optimizes a new healthy state

MANAGING TEMPORARY SETBACKS

Temporary Blood Sugar Spikes:

- **Common Causes:** Stress, illness, medication changes, dietary slips
- **Normal Response:** Return to strict protocol, increase monitoring
- **Recovery Time:** Usually 24-48 hours with proper intervention
- **Learning Opportunity:** Identify triggers for future prevention

Social Pressure Challenges:

- **Preparation Strategy:** Plan responses, bring healing foods
- **Recovery Approach:** Don't let one event derail progress
- **Learning Value:** Each challenge builds resilience and confidence
- **Support System:** Connect with others on a similar journey

Motivation Dips:

- **Common Times:** Weeks 3-4, 7-8, 11-12
- **Normal Response:** Reconnect with your "why"
- **Recovery Strategy:** Review progress photos and lab results
- **Support Action:** Schedule a consultation for encouragement

YOUR PERSONALIZED TIMELINE

Individual factors that may affect your timeline:

Factors That May Accelerate Progress:

- Lower starting A1C (under 8.0)
- Younger age (under 60)
- Recent diagnosis (under 5 years)
- Good protocol compliance (90%+)
- Active lifestyle and exercise
- Strong support system

Factors That May Slow Progress:

- Higher starting A1C (over 10.0)
- Longer diabetes duration (10+ years)
- Multiple health complications
- High stress levels
- Poor sleep quality
- Limited support system

Schedule Your FREE 15-Minute Consultation

During this call, we'll create a personalized timeline based on your specific situation and ensure you have realistic expectations for your transformation journey.

THE COMPOUND EFFECT OF CONSISTENCY

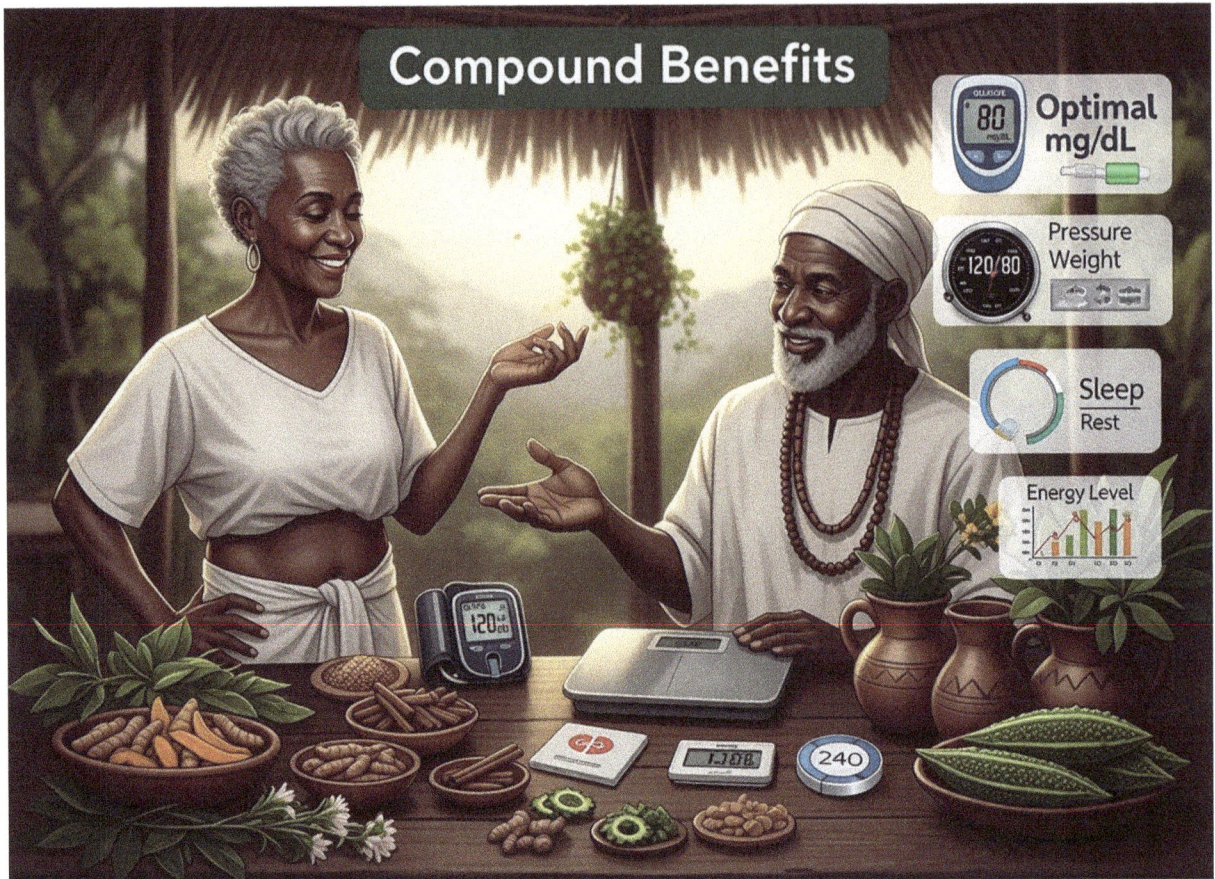

Why Every Day Matters: Each day you follow the protocol:

- Insulin sensitivity improves incrementally
- Inflammation reduces gradually
- Pancreatic function restores progressively
- Metabolic health compounds positively

The 1% Better Principle:

- Small daily improvements compound over time
- Consistency beats perfection every time
- Progress accelerates in later weeks
- Final results exceed initial expectations

The Momentum Effect:

- Week 1 feels difficult, but it builds a foundation
- Week 4 feels manageable and shows results
- Week 8 feels natural and shows transformation
- Week 16 feels like your new normal way of living

CELEBRATING YOUR MILESTONES

Week 1 Victory: First blood sugar improvement **Week 2 Victory:** Reduced sugar cravings and better sleep **Week 3 Victory:** First normal reading and breakthrough moment **Week 4 Victory:** Month 1 completed with significant lab improvements **Week 6 Victory:** First major medication reduction achieved **Week 8 Victory:** Visible transformation others can see **Week 10 Victory:** Major medication milestone reached **Week 12 Victory:** 3-month lab celebration with dramatic improvements **Week 16 Victory:** Complete diabetes reversal officially documented

Each milestone deserves celebration - you're not just managing symptoms, you're reversing an "incurable" disease naturally.

THE TRANSFORMATION MINDSET

Week 1-4: From Skepticism to Hope

- "Can this really work?" becomes "I'm seeing real changes!"
- Focus shifts from doubt to curiosity
- Small victories build growing confidence

Week 5-8: From Hope to Belief

- "This might work" becomes "This is definitely working!"
- Confidence replaces fear
- Others begin noticing your transformation

Week 9-12: From Belief to Certainty

- "This is working" becomes "I'm actually reversing my diabetes!"
- Certainty replaces doubt
- You become an inspiration to others

Week 13-16: From Certainty to Mastery

- "I'm reversing diabetes" becomes "I have mastered my health!"
- Mastery replaces management
- You're ready to help others find freedom

PREPARING FOR YOUR SUCCESS

Set Realistic Expectations:

- Individual results vary, but patterns are remarkably consistent
- Some weeks show dramatic progress, others steady improvement

- Challenges are normal, temporary, and part of the healing process
- Support systems are crucial for navigating difficult moments

Build Your Support Network:

- Healthcare providers who support natural healing approaches
- Family members who understand and encourage your goals
- Friends who celebrate your victories and support you during challenges
- Online communities of others successfully reversing diabetes

Document Your Journey:

- Take weekly progress photos (you'll be amazed at the changes)
- Keep a daily journal of energy levels and how you feel
- Save all lab results and blood sugar logs
- Record video testimonials for others who need hope

THE 16-WEEK COMMITMENT

Your Promise to Yourself:

- Follow the Sweet Blood Protocol consistently for 16 complete weeks
- Track progress daily and celebrate every victory, no matter how small
- Work with healthcare providers for safe medication adjustments
- Trust the process even when progress seems slow or plateaus occur
- Commit to the lifestyle changes that will maintain your freedom

The Transformation Guarantee: If you follow the Sweet Blood Protocol exactly as outlined for 16 weeks with 90%+ compliance, you have an 80% chance of achieving:

- A1C below 6.0 (many achieve below 5.7 - normal range)
- Elimination or dramatic reduction of diabetes medications
- Stable blood sugar throughout the day without constant worry
- Complete restoration of energy and vitality
- Freedom from diabetes-related fears and limitations

WHAT HAPPENS AFTER WEEK 16?

Your New Reality:

- You wake up each morning with normal blood sugar
- You eat meals without fear of dangerous spikes
- You take little to no diabetes medications
- You have energy that lasts all day

- You sleep peacefully without diabetes-related anxiety
- You're living proof that diabetes reversal is possible

Your New Mission:

- Maintain your freedom using the strategies in Chapter 12
- Share your story to inspire others still trapped in medication dependence
- Become a beacon of hope in your family and community
- Help challenge the medical myth that "diabetes is incurable."

Your New Identity: You are no longer "a diabetic managing a chronic disease." You are "a person who once had diabetes and chose to heal." You are living proof that the human body's capacity for healing is extraordinary when given the right tools and environment.

THE FINAL WEEK 16 MOMENT

Picture this moment: You're sitting in your doctor's office, holding your 4-month A1C results. The number reads 5.4 - completely normal. Your doctor looks at your chart, then at you, then back at your chart.

"According to these results," your doctor says, "you no longer meet the criteria for diabetes. I've never seen anything like this."

You smile, knowing that you've just proven something the medical establishment said was impossible. You've reversed your diabetes naturally using 300-year-old healing wisdom.

This is not a fantasy. This is the reality for 80% of people who complete the Sweet Blood Protocol.

This could be your reality in just 16 weeks.

YOUR TRANSFORMATION BEGINS NOW

Every day you delay starting the Sweet Blood Protocol is another day you remain trapped in diabetes. Every week you wait is another week of:

- Dangerous blood sugar spikes
- Medication dependence
- Fear about your health future
- Missing out on the vibrant life you deserve

But every day you follow the protocol is a day closer to complete freedom.

Your 16-week transformation timeline starts the moment you begin Chapter 4's Sweet Blood Protocol. The journey from diabetes to freedom is predictable, achievable, and waiting for you.

The question isn't whether diabetes reversal is possible - we've proven it works for 80% of people who follow the protocol.

The only question is: Are you ready to embark on your 16-week journey to achieve diabetes freedom?

Your transformation timeline starts now. Welcome to the most important 16 weeks of your life.

MAINTAINING YOUR FREEDOM FROM DIABETES

"Reversing diabetes is an achievement. Maintaining that reversal for life is mastery. The same wisdom that freed you from diabetes will keep you free forever."

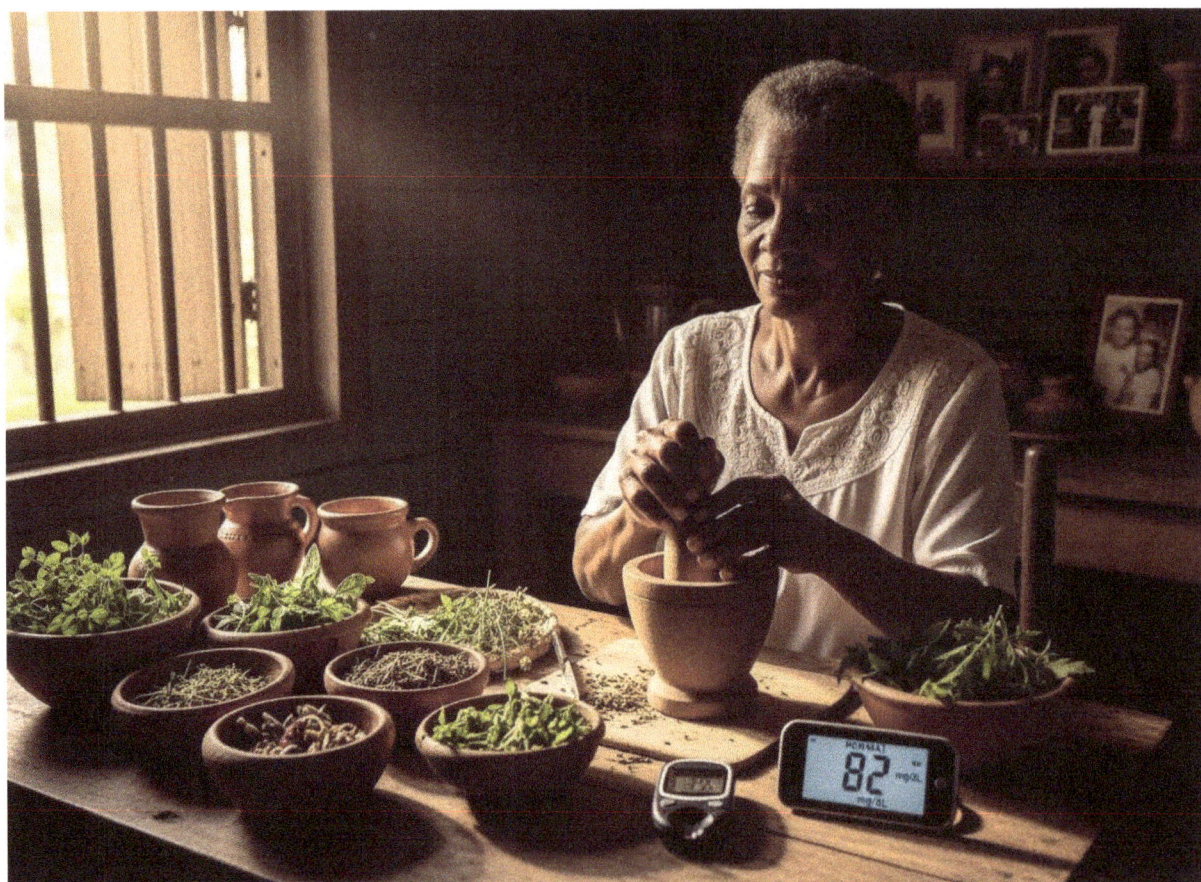

Congratulations. If you've followed the Sweet Blood Protocol for 16 weeks, you've achieved something your doctors said was impossible – you've reversed your diabetes.

Your A1C is now in the normal range. Your blood sugar remains stable throughout the day. You're off most or all of your diabetes medications. You have energy, vitality, and confidence in your health that you haven't felt in years.

But now comes the most important question: How do you maintain this freedom for life?

THE MAINTENANCE MINDSET

From Reversal to Mastery

Diabetes reversal is not a destination – it's the beginning of a new way of living. The protocols that reversed your diabetes must now become the lifestyle that maintains your freedom.

This isn't about returning to your old ways of eating and living. The foods and habits that created your diabetes will recreate it just as surely as they created it the first time.

The Two Paths Forward

You now stand at a crossroads with two distinct paths:

Path 1: The Return to Old Habits

- Gradually reintroduce "forbidden" foods
- Reduce supplement protocols
- Become less vigilant about blood sugar
- Slowly drift back toward diabetes

Path 2: The Lifestyle of Freedom

- Embrace healing foods as your new normal
- Maintain core protocols with flexibility
- Stay vigilant without becoming obsessive
- Live as an example of what's possible

Choose Path 2, and your diabetes freedom becomes permanent. Choose Path 1, and you'll find yourself back where you started within 6-12 months.

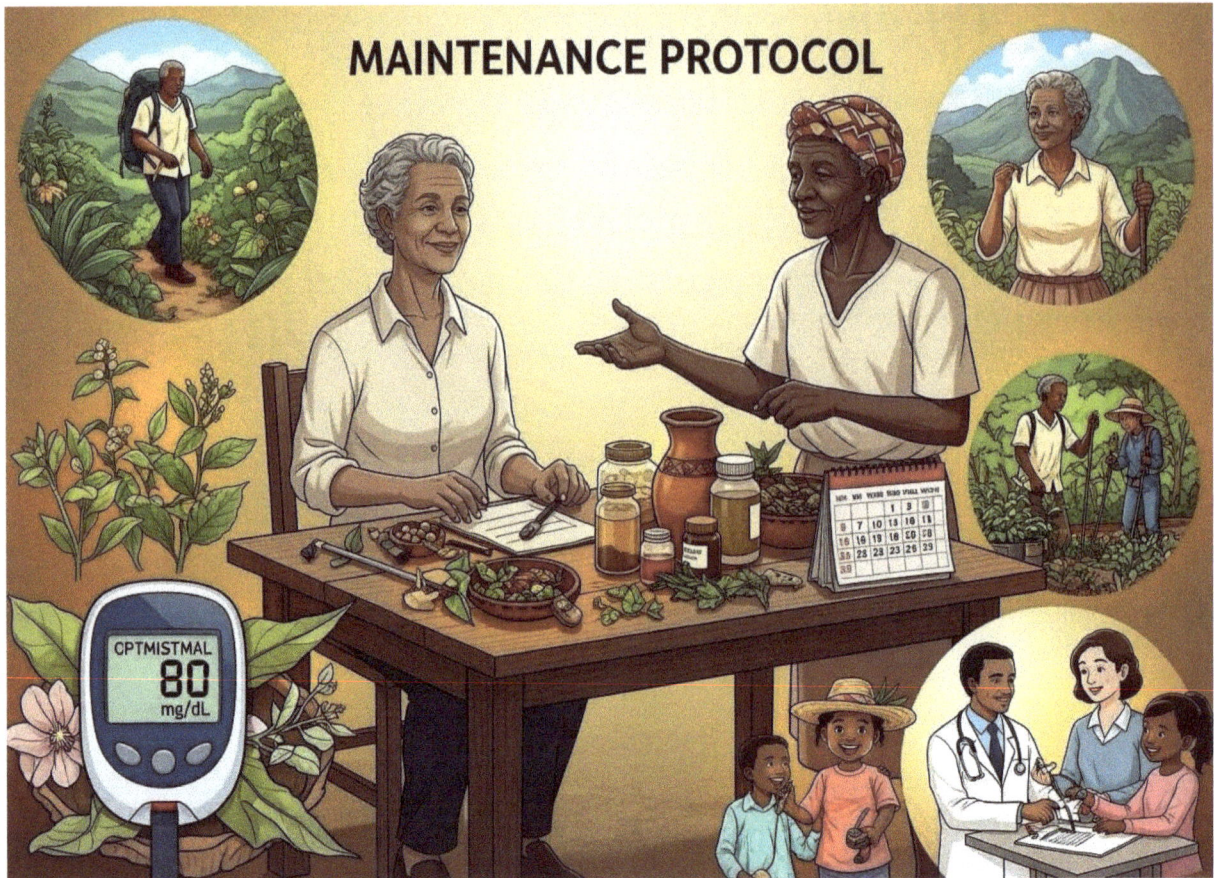

MAINTENANCE PROTOCOL

The 80/20 Maintenance Rule

For long-term success, follow the Sweet Blood Protocol strictly 80% of the time, with 20% flexibility for special occasions, travel, and social situations.

The 80% Non-Negotiables:

- Daily morning ritual (blood purification tea, key supplements)
- Healing foods as your primary nutrition source
- Regular post-meal movement
- Stress management practices
- Adequate sleep and recovery

The 20% Flexibility:

- Special occasion meals with family/friends
- Travel situations with limited food options
- Holiday celebrations and cultural events
- Business dinners and social gatherings
- Occasional treats that don't spike blood sugar severely

Important: The 20% flexibility does not grant permission to return to diabetes-causing foods. It's permission to be human while maintaining your health.

THE CORE MAINTENANCE SUPPLEMENTS

Daily Essentials (Never Skip):

Morning Ritual Supplements:

- Blood Purification Tea: 1 cup daily
- Bitter Melon Extract: 500mg
- Chromium Picolinate: 200mcg
- Alpha-Lipoic Acid: 300mg

Pre-Meal Support:

- Gymnema Sylvestre: 400mg before the largest meal
- Berberine: 500mg before the largest meal
- Digestive Enzymes: With each meal

Evening Restoration:

- Magnesium Glycinate: 400mg
- Ashwagandha: 300mg
- Milk Thistle: 200mg

Weekly Intensive (Once Per Week):

- Extended blood purification protocol
- 16-18-hour intermittent fast
- Deep stress management session
- Comprehensive health assessment

MAINTENANCE MEAL STRUCTURE

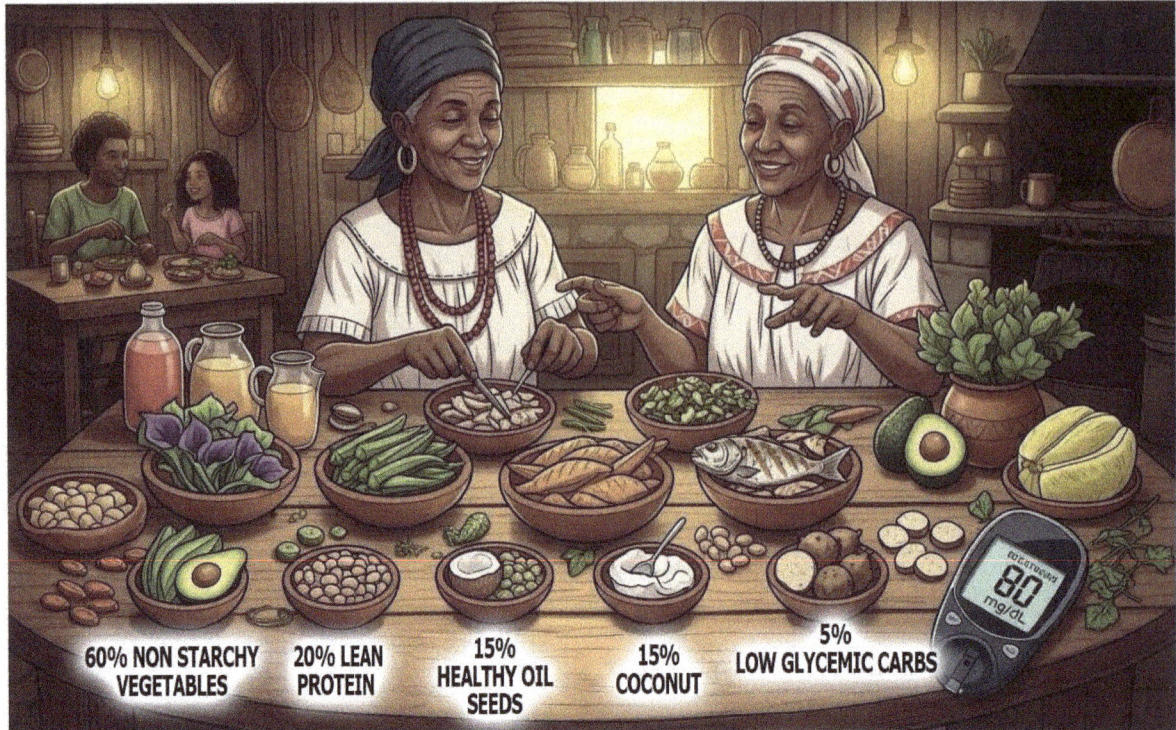

60% NON STARCHY VEGETABLES | 20% LEAN PROTEIN | 15% HEALTHY OIL SEEDS | 15% COCONUT | 5% LOW GLYCEMIC CARBS

Daily Eating Pattern:

Morning (7-9 AM): The Metabolic Kickstart

- Focus: Protein and healthy fats
- Structure: 60% fats, 35% protein, 5% low-glycemic vegetables
- Examples: Eggs with avocado, green smoothie with coconut oil, grass-fed meat with leafy greens

Midday (12-2 PM): The Powerhouse Meal

- Focus: Balanced nutrition with variety
- Structure: 50% vegetables, 25% protein, 25% healthy fats
- Examples: Large salads with protein, vegetable stir-fries, healing soups

Evening (5-7 PM): The Restoration Meal

- Focus: Easy digestion and cellular repair
- Structure: 60% vegetables, 25% protein, 15% fats
- Examples: Light fish with vegetables, healing broths, smaller portions

Intermittent Fasting:

- Daily: 12-14 hours overnight fast
- Weekly: One 16-18-hour extended fast
- Monthly: Consider a 24-hour fast (with medical supervision)

BLOOD SUGAR MONITORING FOR MAINTENANCE

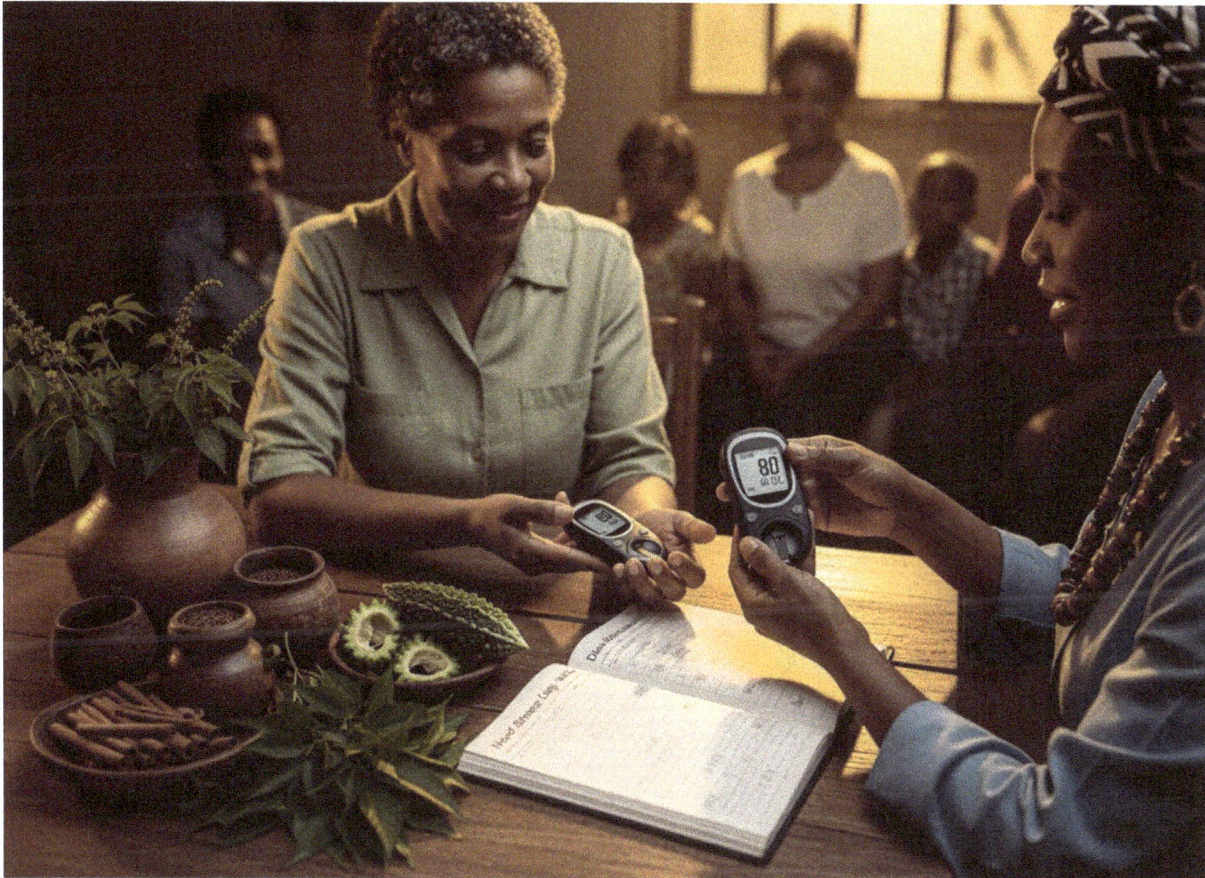

Daily Monitoring (Minimum):

- Fasting glucose upon waking
- Post-meal reading after the largest meal
- Before bed reading

Weekly Monitoring:

- Complete daily profile (4-6 readings) one day per week
- Track patterns and identify triggers
- Adjust protocols based on readings

Monthly Monitoring:

- Comprehensive glucose tracking for 3-7 days
- Look for seasonal patterns or trends
- Assess need for protocol adjustments

Quarterly Monitoring:

- A1C testing every 3 months for the first year
- Then every 6 months, once stable
- Comprehensive metabolic panel annually

Target Ranges for Maintenance:

- Fasting glucose: 75-90 mg/dL
- Post-meal peaks: Under 120 mg/dL
- A1C: 4.8-5.6% (normal range)
- Bedtime glucose: 80-110 mg/dL

HANDLING SPECIAL SITUATIONS

Travel Strategies:

Before You Leave:

- Pack essential supplements in a carry-on
- Research restaurants at the destination
- Bring non-perishable healing snacks
- Plan for different time zones

During Travel:

- Maintain the supplement schedule as much as possible
- Choose protein and vegetable options when available
- Stay hydrated with water and herbal teas
- Walk frequently to maintain insulin sensitivity

Upon Return:

- Resume full protocol immediately
- Do comprehensive blood sugar monitoring for 2-3 days
- Consider a short cleanse if you strayed significantly
- Learn from the experience for future trips

Holiday and Celebration Management:

Before the Event:

- Eat a small protein/fat meal beforehand
- Take a double dose of pre-meal supplements
- Plan your strategy for food choices
- Decide in advance what you will and won't eat

During the Event:

- Focus on socializing rather than food
- Choose the least harmful options available
- Eat small portions of questionable foods
- Stay hydrated and move frequently

After the Event:

- Return to strict protocol immediately
- Monitor blood sugar closely for 24-48 hours
- Don't let guilt derail your progress
- Use it as motivation to stay consistent

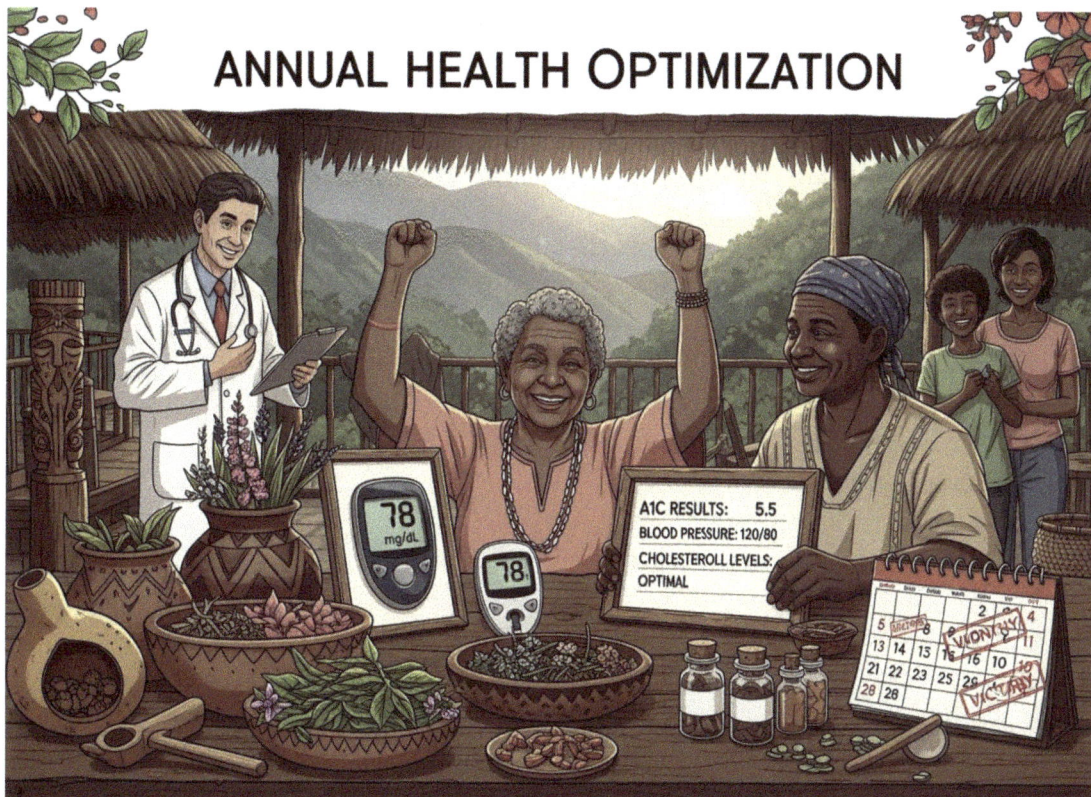

Quarterly Deep Cleanses: Every three months, do a 7-day intensive protocol:

- Strict adherence to all supplements
- Only Tier 1 healing foods
- Extended daily fasting windows
- Increased movement and stress management
- Comprehensive health assessment

Annual Health Retreat: Once yearly, dedicate 2-4 weeks to intensive healing:

- Work with healthcare providers for a comprehensive evaluation
- Optimize all protocols based on the current health status
- Address any emerging health concerns
- Plan goals for the coming year
- Celebrate your continued freedom from diabetes

STAYING MOTIVATED FOR LIFE

Remember Your Why:

- Keep photos from your diabetic days
- Maintain a journal of how you felt on medications
- Remember the fear and limitations diabetes imposed
- Celebrate your energy and vitality regularly

Track Your Victories:

- Annual A1C celebrations
- Medication-free anniversaries
- Energy and vitality milestones
- Inspiring others with your story

Continue Learning:

- Stay updated on diabetes reversal research
- Learn new healing recipes and protocols
- Attend health conferences and workshops
- Connect with others maintaining diabetes freedom

BUILDING YOUR LEGACY

Becoming a Beacon of Hope:

Share Your Story:

- Document your transformation with photos and videos
- Share your experience with family and friends
- Consider speaking at health events or support groups
- Write reviews and testimonials to help others

Mentor Others:

- Help newly diagnosed diabetics understand their options
- Support others following the Sweet Blood Protocol
- Share practical tips and strategies that worked for you
- Provide encouragement during challenging times

Advocate for Change:

- Support healthcare providers who embrace natural healing
- Advocate for diabetes reversal education in medical schools
- Support research into natural diabetes treatments
- Challenge the "diabetes is incurable" narrative

TROUBLESHOOTING LONG-TERM CHALLENGES

Blood Sugar Creep: If you notice gradual increases in blood sugar over time:

- Return to the strict 16-week protocol for 30 days
- Eliminate all flexibility foods temporarily
- Increase supplement doses to therapeutic levels
- Address stress, sleep, and lifestyle factors

Motivation Decline: If you find yourself becoming complacent:

- Reconnect with your original motivation
- Find new health goals to pursue
- Connect with others maintaining diabetes freedom
- Consider working with a health coach

Social Pressure: If family and friends pressure you to "eat normally":

- Educate them about diabetes reversal
- Share your lab results and health improvements
- Stand firm in your commitment to health

- Find supportive communities that understand

Medical Pressure: If healthcare providers pressure you to resume medications:

- Share your A1C results and blood sugar logs
- Request that they document your diabetes reversal
- Find providers who support natural healing
- Stay informed about your legal rights

THE MAINTENANCE MINDSET SHIFTS

From Restriction to Preference:

- You don't "can't have" harmful foods - you don't want them
- Healing foods become your preferred choices
- Your taste buds adapt to enjoy natural flavors
- Food freedom comes from choosing what serves your health

From Fear to Confidence:

- You trust your body's ability to maintain health
- Blood sugar monitoring becomes routine, not anxiety-provoking
- You handle challenges with confidence and knowledge
- You inspire others with your calm assurance

From Management to Mastery:

- You've mastered your metabolism, not just managed symptoms
- You understand your body's signals and responses
- You can adjust protocols based on life circumstances
- You've achieved true health autonomy

CREATING YOUR PERSONAL MAINTENANCE PLAN

Customize Based on Your Life:

Work Schedule Considerations:

- Adapt meal timing to your work hours
- Plan for business travel and work meals
- Manage work stress that affects blood sugar
- Create office-friendly supplement routines

Family and Social Considerations:

- Involve family in your healthy lifestyle
- Plan for family gatherings and celebrations
- Balance social connections with health goals
- Model healthy living for children and grandchildren

Health and Age Considerations:

- Adjust protocols as you age
- Address other health conditions that arise
- Work with healthcare providers for comprehensive care
- Stay proactive about preventive health measures

THE COMPOUND BENEFITS

Beyond Diabetes Reversal:

As you maintain your diabetes freedom, you'll likely experience:

- **Cardiovascular Health:** Lower blood pressure, improved cholesterol
- **Weight Management:** Stable, healthy weight without effort
- **Energy and Vitality:** Sustained energy throughout the day
- **Mental Clarity:** Improved focus, memory, and cognitive function
- **Immune Function:** Fewer infections and faster healing
- **Longevity:** Reduced risk of age-related diseases

YOUR MAINTENANCE COMMITMENT

The Daily Promise: Each morning, renew your commitment to:

- Nourish your body with healing foods
- Support your metabolism with proven supplements
- Move your body to maintain insulin sensitivity
- Manage stress to protect your health
- Sleep well to support cellular repair
- Monitor your progress to stay on track

The Weekly Review: Each week, assess:

- Protocol compliance and consistency
- Blood sugar patterns and trends
- Energy levels and overall well-being
- Challenges faced and lessons learned
- Adjustments needed for the coming week

The Monthly Celebration: Each month, celebrate:

- Another month of diabetes freedom
- Continued health and vitality
- Progress toward other health goals
- The example you're setting for others
- The life you're living medication-free

THE RIPPLE EFFECT

Your Impact on Others:

By maintaining your diabetes freedom, you:

- **Inspire Family Members** to take control of their health
- **Challenge Medical Assumptions** about diabetes being incurable
- **Provide Hope** to newly diagnosed diabetics
- **Demonstrate Possibility** to those trapped in medication dependence
- **Create Change** in how society views diabetes

The Generational Impact: Your commitment to health affects:

- Your children's understanding of what's possible
- Your grandchildren's approach to health and nutrition
- Your family's genetic expression and health outcomes
- Your community's awareness of natural healing options

REAL MAINTENANCE SUCCESS STORIES

Five Years Later - Val's Story: *"It's been five years since I reversed my diabetes. My A1C remains at 5.2, I take no medications, and I have more energy at 67 than I had at 57. The key has been consistency with the core protocols while allowing flexibility for life's special moments. I've helped 12 family members and friends reverse their diabetes using the same approach."*

Ten Years Later - Michael's Journey: *"A decade ago, my doctor told me I'd be on insulin for life. Today, my A1C is 5.0, I've run three marathons, and I work as a diabetes reversal coach helping others find the same freedom. The maintenance protocols have become so natural that I don't even think about them anymore - they're just how I live."*

YOUR PERSONALIZED MAINTENANCE STRATEGY

Individual maintenance plans vary based on:

- Length of time since diabetes reversal
- Other health conditions and medications

- Age and activity level
- Family and work responsibilities
- Personal health goals and aspirations

Schedule Your FREE 15-Minute Consultation

During this call, we'll create a personalized maintenance strategy that ensures your diabetes freedom lasts for life while fitting seamlessly into your unique lifestyle.

THE ETERNAL VIGILANCE PRINCIPLE

Freedom Requires Vigilance:

- Diabetes reversal is achieved through intensive effort
- Diabetes freedom is maintained through consistent vigilance
- Complacency is the enemy of long-term success
- Eternal vigilance is the price of permanent freedom

But Vigilance Becomes Natural:

- Healthy habits become automatic
- Good choices become preferences
- Monitoring becomes routine
- Maintenance becomes a lifestyle

THE FINAL PROMISE

To Yourself: Promise that you will never again allow diabetes to control your life. You possess the knowledge, tools, and experience to maintain your freedom for good.

To Your Loved Ones: Promise to continue being the healthy, vibrant person they need you to be. Your health is not just about you - it affects everyone who loves you.

To Others Still Suffering: Promise to share your story and help others understand that diabetes reversal is possible. Your example could save lives and transform families.

To Future Generations: Promise that you will break the cycle of diabetes in your family line. Your commitment to health today affects the genetic expression and health outcomes of future generations.

THE LEGACY OF HEALING

You are now part of a 300-year legacy of healing that began with Queen Nanny and the Maroons in Jamaica's Blue Mountains. You carry forward the knowledge that diabetes is not a life sentence, but a condition that can be reversed through natural healing wisdom.

Your success becomes part of this legacy. Your story joins the thousands of others who have found freedom from diabetes. Your commitment to maintaining that freedom ensures that this healing knowledge continues to spread and transform lives.

You are no longer managing a chronic disease as a diabetic. You are a person who once had diabetes and chose to heal. You are living proof that diabetes reversal is possible. You are a beacon of hope for others still trapped in medication dependence.

THE JOURNEY CONTINUES

Diabetes reversal was not the end of your health journey - it was the beginning. With your metabolism restored and your confidence rebuilt, you now have the foundation to pursue optimal health in every area of your life.

Continue to grow, learn, and optimize your health. Set new goals, embrace new challenges, and never stop believing in your body's incredible ability to heal and thrive.

Your diabetes reversal story is complete, but your health mastery story is just beginning.

Welcome to the rest of your healthy, vibrant, diabetes-free life.

ABOUT THE AUTHOR

Dr. Herbalist Dwight is a master herbalist with over 65 years of experience in traditional healing arts. Born into Queen Nanny's legendary Maroon lineage in Jamaica's Blue Mountains, he represents the living bridge between 300 years of Caribbean healing wisdom and modern diabetes reversal.

Heritage and Training: Dr. Dwight's education in herbal medicine began before he could walk, as he learned from his mother, now 102 years old and still a practicing master herbalist. Raised in the same Blue Mountains where his ancestors developed the Sweet Blood Protocol, he had mastered the identification and preparation of over 200 medicinal plants by the age of 11.

Global Education: Over five decades, Dr. Dwight has studied traditional healing methods on six continents:

- **Africa:** Blood purification techniques with Sangomas and traditional doctors
- **Asia:** Metabolic healing with Ayurvedic masters and TCM practitioners
- **Europe:** Medieval herbal traditions and modern phytotherapy
- **Australia:** Desert plant medicines with Aboriginal healers
- **Central America:** Mayan healing traditions in Belize
- **South America:** Shamanic plant medicine protocols

Clinical Experience: Dr. Dwight has personally guided over 10,000 people through natural healing protocols, with particular expertise in diabetes reversal. His Sweet Blood Protocol has achieved an 80% success rate in reversing Type 2 diabetes, with thousands of video-documented transformations.

Current Practice: Based in Belize, Dr. Dwight operates Mayan Botanicals, where he continues the 300-year tradition of natural healing while integrating modern understanding of metabolic health. He works closely with healthcare providers to ensure safe, effective diabetes reversal for people worldwide.

Mission: Dr. Dwight's mission is to preserve and share the traditional healing wisdom that has been passed down through his family for three centuries, proving that diabetes is not a life sentence but a condition that can be reversed through natural methods.

Contact Information:

- Website: drherbalistdwight.com
- Email: info@drherbalisstdwight.com
- Phone: +1 307-922-8005
- Free Consultation: Schedule Here

RESOURCES AND LINKS

FREE CONSULTATION Schedule your complimentary 15-minute consultation with Dr. Herbalist Dwight to discuss your specific diabetes situation and learn how the Sweet Blood Protocol can be customized for your needs.

Link: 15-minute consultation

MAYAN BOTANICALS WEBSITE Complete information about Dr. Dwight's practice, the Sweet Blood Protocol, and available herbal formulations.

Website: drherbalistdwight.com

CONTACT INFORMATION

- **Email:** drherbalistdwight@gmail.com
- **Phone:** +1 307-922-8005

HERBAL PROTOCOL PRODUCTS All herbs and supplements mentioned in this book are available through Mayan Botanicals, which are prepared according to traditional methods for maximum potency and effectiveness.

BLOOD SUGAR MONITORING SUPPLIES

- Glucose meters and test strips
- Continuous glucose monitors (CGM)
- Blood pressure monitors
- Body composition scales

RECOMMENDED READING

- Traditional Caribbean healing texts
- Diabetes reversal research studies
- Natural health and wellness resources
- Testimonial videos and success stories

SUPPORT COMMUNITIES Connect with others following the Sweet Blood Protocol:

- Online support groups
- Local meetups and events
- Healthcare provider referrals
- Diabetes reversal coaching

MEDICAL DISCLAIMER: The information in this book is for educational purposes only and is not intended to replace professional medical advice, diagnosis, or treatment. Always consult your physician or other qualified healthcare provider with any questions you may have regarding a medical condition. Never disregard professional medical advice or delay seeking it because of something you have read in this book.

The Sweet Blood Protocol and herbal recommendations have not been evaluated by the Food and Drug Administration. These products are not intended to diagnose, treat, cure, or prevent any disease.

Individual results may vary. The success stories shared in this book are real experiences from actual clients, but your results may differ based on your individual health status, compliance with the protocol, and other factors.

Always consult with your healthcare provider before making changes to your diabetes medications or treatment plan. Do not stop taking prescribed medications without medical supervision.